Praise for *Ready for My Surgery*

"Having surgery is just like embarking on a journey to a foreign country. Savvy travellers minimize misadventures by fully preparing for their trips. *Ready for My Surgery* is *the* ultimate travel guide, including an essential packing list and useful (medical) language translator. Don't plan a hospital procedure without it!"

DR. LUCIE FILTEAU Anesthesiologist, The Ottawa Hospital; Chair, Patient Safety Committee, Canadian Anesthesiologists' Society

"There is a growing understanding that patients themselves, as well as their families, constitute a vital component of how quality and safety in the healthcare system is achieved. What this means for patients is that how active a role they take within the healthcare they receive can often have a significant impact on how effective that care is. *Ready for My Surgery* supports patients to take control of their own care. Author Patrick J. Nellis leverages his substantial experience and expertise to empower people with knowledge about their surgery, and offers them strategies to build inclusive partnerships with their healthcare providers. Nellis' thoughtful and straightforward writing delivers insights that are sure to help improve the way many patients and families experience surgery."

DR. ANDREW WEST EdD, FCSRT; CEO, Canadian Society of Respiratory Therapists

"What a fantastic book. It covers just about everything you'd ever want to know. My father had cardiac bypass surgery this last spring and I gave the book to him as a gift. He was an airline pilot for his entire career and is someone used to being well informed and in control of his circumstances. This book helped him prepare for the surgery and that preparation helped him feel more in control during the entire process. Thanks, from both me and my dad!"

KEVIN TAYLOR RRT, MBA

"Patrick J. Nellis' insights are a welcome change from the limited information most patients receive before they have surgery. *Ready for My Surgery* is a wonderful book that will assist many patients in answering questions that are often misunderstood or not given much thought."

DONNA PENNER Patients for Patient Safety Canada

"Congratulations to Patrick J. Nellis for writing this book. It is extensive in its scope. It is a great resource and contains a wealth of information for anyone wishing to understand what transpires in the perioperative period."

DR. PAUL S. TUMBER Director of Education, Chronic Pain, Assistant Professor of Anesthesiology, University of Toronto

"Although I am not a neophyte when it comes to undergoing surgeries, I still found *Ready for My Surgery* to be a great source of information. This book will help anyone who is facing an upcoming surgery to go into the OR feeling better informed and better prepared. Thank you for sharing your expertise and experience."

LOUISE WOODS Canadian patient

"At the Canadian Patient Safety Institute, we know that every 1 minute and 18 seconds a person receiving care in hospital or in their home is unintentionally harmed by the healthcare system. Everyone has a role to play in keeping patients safe, including the patient themselves and their family. Patrick J. Nellis' book is an excellent resource to assist patients and their families to prepare for surgery, helping them understand what to expect and what they and those caring for them must do to provide a safe experience. I would highly recommend this book to anyone undergoing a surgical procedure. A clear, instructive and compelling read that will prepare you well for your surgical journey!"

CHRIS POWER CEO, Canadian Patient Safety Institute

"Healthcare can be an intimidating environment from the side of the patient, with too many patients being afraid of asking questions and taking control of their experience. Patrick J. Nellis has written the perfect easy-to-read guide from an insider's view. He's heard all the questions, and he clearly knows how to navigate the system in a healthy, empowering manner. As fellow healthcare professionals, we can assure you that he has done a brilliant job of decoding the experience, giving great tips on how to make the most of a surgical experience. We highly recommend this resource and can't wait to see it literally change the experience for patients everywhere."

SCOT JONES BA, RRT, RRT-ACCS; Respiratory Therapist and author
DANA OAKES BA, RRT, RRT-NPS; Respiratory Therapist and author

"As patients, we trust our healthcare team during one of the most vulnerable events in our lives: surgery. However, we know from personal experience, research and media reports that surgery is not risk-free. Preventable incidents like wrong site surgery and surgical site infections have profound effects on patients and families. This book helps us understand the surgical process and equips us with knowledge, a fundamental tool to strengthen patient safety. Knowledge helps us prepare properly for surgery, ask the right questions, keep an eye out for risks and speak up when we have concerns. It can even help us recover without setbacks. In *Ready for My Surgery*, Patrick J. Nellis shows us both the big picture and a detailed dive into evidence when needed. As contributors, Patients for Patient Safety Canada would like to see it in the hands of all pre-surgical patients and their families so that everyone has a safe surgical experience."

PATIENTS FOR PATIENT SAFETY CANADA

"On behalf of the RTSO Executive Committee, we are proud to endorse *Ready for My Surgery*. This book is a key element of a new surgical patient engagement program, designed to support surgical patients through engagement, education and empowerment. As a past-President of the RTSO, we are especially proud of Patrick J. Nellis' ongoing contribution toward excellent patient care through this book and throughout his career. Expertly written for patients, *Ready for My Surgery* informatively reviews various care aspects surrounding the surgical experience. The book and program ultimately empower patients to take control of their health through becoming informed and engaged members of their healthcare team."

RESPIRATORY THERAPY SOCIETY OF ONTARIO

"As a healthcare provider reviewing this book, I found it to provide enlightening insight into the patient journey. It reminds clinicians that better outcomes are possible with patients who are actively involved in their health and stresses the importance of working and learning collaboratively. It reminds us that empathy and compassion play vital roles in the patient experience."

SHAWNA MACDONALD RRT, FCSRT; Director, Respiratory Therapy Society of Ontario

READY FOR MY SURGERY

PATRICK J. NELLIS

READY
for My
SURGERY

Be INFORMED, stay SAFE
and take CONTROL during your
journey through surgery

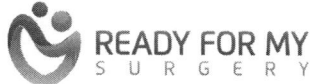

Copyright © 2020 by Patrick J. Nellis

All rights reserved. No part of this book may be reproduced, stored in a retrieval system or transmitted, in any form or by any means, without the prior written consent of the publisher or a licence from The Canadian Copyright Licensing Agency (Access Copyright). For a copyright licence, visit www.accesscopyright.ca or call toll free to 1-800-893-5777.

Every reasonable effort has been made to contact the copyright holders for work reproduced in this book.

Some names and identifying details have been changed to protect the privacy of individuals.

This book is not intended as a substitute for the medical advice of physicians. The reader should regularly consult a physician in matters relating to his/her health and particularly with respect to any symptoms that may require diagnosis or medical attention.

ISBN 978-1-9992441-1-8 (paperback)
ISBN 978-1-9992441-0-1 (ebook)

Published by Ready for My Surgery
www.readyformysurgery.com

Produced by Page Two
www.pagetwo.com

www.readyformysurgery.com

To Tanya, Nicole and Ryan—for your love and support as this book grew from dream into reality.

To the patients and families who have inspired me as they braved the path through surgery.

CONTENTS

FOREWORD BY CLAUDE LAFLAMME
MD, FRCPC, MHSC xiii

PREFACE xv

INTRODUCTION 1
HOW TO USE THIS BOOK 5
QUICK SUMMARY 7

1 Scheduled for Surgery 15

2 Hospitals & Surgery Centres 35

3 The Day of Surgery 51

4 Recovering from Surgery 91

5 Giving Feedback & Giving Back 131

ACKNOWLEDGEMENTS 141

APPENDIX A 143
Ready for My Surgery Checklist

APPENDIX B 149
Medical Tests

APPENDIX C 155
Monitoring in the Operating Room

APPENDIX D 161
Resources

INDEX 163

FOREWORD

IT IS BOTH a pleasure and an honour to have the opportunity to write the foreword to *Ready for My Surgery*.

Patient education and engagement is an invaluable element of modern medicine. However, only recently has its importance been recognized. Over my 30-year career of practicing anesthesia, I have witnessed the evolution of doctor-patient relationships. Decades ago, patients were reluctant to learn too much about potential complications of their surgery, as the information was perceived to be more anxiety-causing than informative. Since then, technology has revolutionized how we get our information, and has made that information readily available. This abundance of information has encouraged a more meaningful, two-way conversation between patients and healthcare providers. Nowadays, a substantial percentage of patients are informed on the various treatment options offered to them—they want to participate in a decision-making process that will pave the way to an optimal treatment plan. Once decisions are made, it is imperative that patients have access to the comprehensive information that will guide them on the contributions they can make to improve the safety of their care.

This is what author Patrick J. Nellis is offering you in this book. For as long as I have known Patrick, he has been volunteering his time in various capacities in order to improve healthcare safety. Patrick worked as a clinician in operating rooms for many years, and his wealth of clinical experience and dedication to patient safety have led to the creation of this great work. Patrick observed firsthand the anxiety that patients experience in anticipation of their surgery. Furthermore, it has been demonstrated that adequate patient education before surgery decreases anxiety and is associated with improved outcomes.

I can personally testify to the power of knowledge about one's own medical condition, and compliance with instruction and self-management before and after surgery. In 2014, I had major surgery. Being an anesthesiologist and the chair of Enhanced Recovery Canada, I knew the risks of surgery very well, but I also had knowledge on how to engage in my own care. When I was recovering, my loved ones asked me how anxious I had been right before my surgery. They knew that I was well aware of the details of the procedure, and its benefits and risks. The truth is that I was not anxious. I had done my due diligence and complied with the instructions. I felt at peace because I had mentally prepared myself for the recovery phase, I trusted my team, and I had done what I had to do to set myself up for a good outcome.

With this book in your hands, you are about to embark on a journey of self-empowerment. *Ready for My Surgery* is a comprehensive approach that will give you the tools you need to truly engage in your own care. The book is written in simple terms, with chapters that follow the various stages of your surgical journey, from before surgery to rehabilitation. You will learn how to prepare yourself before surgery to minimize the risk of complications, and to recover faster.

Ready for My Surgery is a timely book that aligns with a new healthcare trend—one that is moving toward patient empowerment in a patient-centred system.

CLAUDE LAFLAMME MD, FRCPC, MHSC
Chair, Enhanced Recovery Canada
Assistant Professor, University of Toronto

PREFACE

WHEN I BEGAN writing this book a few years ago, my focus was to help alleviate the anxiety I saw in so many patients before their surgery and help them feel more in control. While this is still important to me and a significant part of what this book delivers, I felt the need to add a few words these years later to share a larger vision of what I believe the patient experience should be.

Through the process of writing, researching and talking to patients and healthcare providers, I've come to understand something that few patients are likely to know—the actions you take (or don't) as a patient can have a direct and profound impact on the outcome of your surgery.

Surgery has enough risk. Simply showing up on the day of your operation and hoping for the best can introduce more, avoidable risks. This is a challenge because most people have no idea. I'd like to change that.

I'd like you to think of yourself as a member of your healthcare team, not just a passive recipient of its care. If you think of yourself in this way, you'll now appreciate that you have a role to play. As with any team, the better each team member understands and fulfills his or her role—and understands the role of each of their fellow team members—the more effective the team will be in achieving its objective. In this case, the objective is a safe surgery with the desired outcome.

You can't control everything, but you can control your part. This book was written to give you the knowledge, tools and insights to help you engage with your healthcare team. It will help you and your loved ones take control of your health and healthcare. Through the process of empowering yourself as a patient, you can feel confident that you are well prepared for each step of your journey through surgery.

Since beginning my work to improve patient safety and engagement, I've had the experience of being present for a loved one in need of urgent surgery for a troubling condition. As with all experiences in life, this broadened my perspective. I have a heightened appreciation of the important role that family, friends and caregivers have in supporting and advocating for patients. Sometimes, patients find themselves in a position where they must rely completely on those at their bedside to be their voice. This is a tremendous responsibility. As such, I see this book to be as applicable for family and friends as it is for patients.

I expect a future in healthcare where we ask more of our patients and their families. We'll ask for a partnership. If our common goal is to improve outcomes for patients and reduce risk, why wouldn't we? I hope this is the future you experience.

Change takes time and persistence. I commend you for taking this time to invest in your health—you are serving yourself well while helping our healthcare system move in the right direction. Know that there are many individuals and organizations that will persist on your behalf to usher in this vision of a partnership between patients and their care providers. We're in this together. Let's continue on with these thoughts in mind and embrace the journey ahead.

INTRODUCTION

BEING A PATIENT isn't easy. Having an operation isn't easy either. I've spent most of my career working with people in your situation. Throughout my years working in the Operating Room (OR), there was one thing I found in great abundance—apprehensive patients quietly waiting their turn to be brought into the mysterious Operating Room.

While it isn't mysterious or frightening to the hospital staff that work there each day, to the outsider—the patient—the anticipation of entering this environment can bring about varying degrees of anxiety.

This anxious anticipation follows people into the Operating Room. Seeing the inside of the OR for the first time can be intimidating for anyone, let alone for the person lying on the surgical table. Many are overwhelmed by the numerous masked healthcare professionals moving about and the flurry of activity that happens to and around them.

The stress that is provoked by this situation has consequences.

Stress hormones rage through many patients as they lay in the OR awaiting "something" to happen to them. Heart rate and blood pressure can be elevated (and usually are). This can even make getting an intravenous (IV) catheter more difficult—no fun at the best of times!

Is there a way to alleviate some of this stress?

Can a sense of vulnerability be replaced with a sense of empowerment?

I believe so.

I've seen firsthand how anxiety is lessened when a person going for surgery knows a little about what to expect. Some want to know everything. Others want to know as little as possible (that's right, let's just get it over with!).

Regardless of your interest in surgery, there's actually much more to your hospital visit than the activities in the OR. In fact, the majority of your time in hospital will be spent before and after surgery.

My goal with you is to knock down that anxiety by arming you with the right mix of information, support and encouragement. Here are some key things we'll tackle together:

- How to get *truly* prepared for your surgery (and why it's important)
- The steps to take to set yourself up for success (I'll give you the tools to do it)
- Your flow through the hospital—from admission to discharge
- What exactly goes on inside an Operating Room when you're asleep
- Insights into the experience of having an anesthetic—falling asleep, waking up and pain control (for a lot of people, this is the scary bit)
- The roles of the people looking after you
- How you should *expect* to participate in your care
- The emotions you may experience (and what to do with them)
- The systems in place to help keep you safe
- The help that is available for your transition home
- The opportunities available to find support from others that have been in your shoes and ways to share your experience (hint: www.readyformysurgery.com)

The sincere appreciation I received from patients as I supported them in and around the time of their surgery was not only a very fulfilling part of my work at the beside, but also a sign that it matters. Reassurance and compassion to those feeling vulnerable and anxious is a wonderful act offered every day by many working in the field of healthcare. Yet while this is true, time is one of the greatest constraints on healthcare professionals today. This places a limitation on how well a patient can be informed just before surgery. The state of mind of those about to have an operation (nervous!) also makes the time just before surgery less than ideal for the flow of information about their care to be consumed and processed effectively.

Surgery is an aspect of healthcare that affects so many yet remains largely a mystery. This book was written to give you an opportunity to acquire a new level of insight into what it means to be an informed patient. If you or a loved one is scheduled for surgery, the knowledge you will acquire here will empower you to be an active participant in your healthcare, to ask questions and to understand that you are the most important part of your care.

The day of surgery is a difficult time to start asking questions, though it is when most people do. This book will answer many questions before they arise and will help friends and family understand their role during this time.

Read on—find the support you need, empower yourself and become an informed and confident consumer of healthcare.

HOW TO USE THIS BOOK

MOST PEOPLE WANT to be prepared for their surgery. Not everyone wants the same amount of information, though. To support these differences, there are two ways to use this book:

1. Quick Summary

This is a brief, point-form summary containing only the key pieces of information you'll need to know. This section will give you the basics. If you'd like to know a little more after reading the Quick Summary, simply flip to the corresponding chapter of the book.

2. Full Book

This book is full of stories, important messages and Insider Tips gained through years of experience and research. If you would like to benefit from this to ensure you are well informed and prepared for your operation, enjoy the book cover-to-cover.

Not sure which is best for you?

Try starting with the Quick Summary to familiarize yourself with the content. To learn more and become better prepared to fufill the role you're meant to play, Chapter 1 is waiting for you.

QUICK SUMMARY

Chapter 1 Summary—Scheduled for Surgery

Essential Information

Your Role — Understanding your role as a patient and being prepared to manage your health and healthcare has been linked to better health outcomes

Your Emotions — When managing your thoughts and emotions related to surgery, acceptance and gratitude are powerful allies

Your Health — If you have any chronic (long-term) health conditions, being properly prepared for surgery means having a basic understanding of each condition, the impact they have on your well-being, how to effectively manage them and how to know that each condition is stable

Your Actions — Your actions before surgery can impact your ability to recover—Enhanced Recovery After Surgery (ERAS) is a program that brings together the key actions that improve your ability to recover from an operation; counselling, proper nutrition and physical activity are essential components of your recovery

Your Smoking — If you smoke, quitting for as long as possible before surgery has a significant impact on your overall health and numerous benefits supporting your recovery from surgery—this is a perfect opportunity to quit for good and the resources available to help have never been greater

Your Tool — Print and use your Ready for My Surgery Checklist—this is an essential tool to help you organize the important information you'll need to keep track of and communicate to your healthcare team (found in Appendix A)

Your Preparation — Be well prepared for your Pre-Admission Clinic visit by completing your Ready for My Surgery Checklist ahead of time—this will allow you to be clear on the questions you want to ask of the anesthesiologist or nurse at the clinic, rather than simply hoping you have answers to their questions and missing the opportunity to ask questions of your own

Your Tests — There are a variety of possible medical tests that may be required of you—x-ray, CT scan, MRI, ultrasound, endoscopy, ECG, pulmonary function tests and blood work (descriptions of each can be found in Appendix B).

Key Takeaways from Chapter 1

- Understand your state of health
- Learn how you can influence the outcome of your surgery
- Get organized using your Ready for My Surgery Checklist

Chapter 2 Summary—Hospitals & Surgery Centres

Essential Information

Your Visit — Find out the type of facility you'll be visiting for your surgery (University Teaching Hospital, Community Hospital or Ambulatory Surgery Centre), understand the differences, prepare your travel and arrive prepared

Your Checklist — Identify the sections of your Ready for My Surgery Checklist that you can't complete on your own and if needed, make appointments with the people who can help you find the answers

Your Healthcare Professionals — You'll be working with many different professionals during your journey through surgery—by learning a little about them, you can better understand how and when each can support your healthcare

Your Flow Through the Hospital — Once in hospital, each stage of your operation brings you to a different department—Surgical Reception → Pre-Operative Area → Operating Room → Post-Anesthetic Care Unit (and sometimes to the Hospital Ward or Intensive Care Unit)—understanding this flow and the function of each space will allow you to anticipate and be at ease with each transition

Key Takeaways from Chapter 2

- Prepare for your visit to the hospital/Surgery Centre
- Understand your travel to and movement within the facility
- Learn a little about who you'll be working with

Chapter 3 Summary—The Day of Surgery

Essential Information

Your Night Before Surgery — On the night before surgery: 1) review your Ready for My Surgery Checklist; 2) review instructions from your surgeon/anesthesiologist/Pre-Admission Clinic nurse; 3) connect with the person going with you to the hospital; 4) relax in a healthy way; 5) sleep well

Your Fasting — Follow the fasting guidelines given to you—avoid dehydration by drinking clear fluids until the allowed deadline

Your Moments Before Surgery — The Pre-Operative Area (the place you'll wait before going into the Operating Room) will come with many questions and interactions with hospital staff—your *active participation here is critical* to avoid mistakes and misunderstandings

Understanding Blood Transfusions — If your surgery has the potential for you to receive a blood transfusion, understanding the risks and benefits is important for you to make an informed decision

Correct Patient, Correct Site, Correct Procedure — Important guidelines from the World Health Organization (WHO) are in place to reduce the risk of an error in communication about your surgery—you are expected to be an active participant in making sure **You** get the **Correct Procedure** on the **Correct Site** of your body

Your Anesthetic — Your anesthesia care may be provided by one or more professionals that can include physician and non-physician care providers—be prepared to have the most in-depth conversations about your state of health with your Anesthesia Care Team

Delays & Cancellations — Be aware that there is always a small but real risk that your surgery can be delayed or cancelled, even as you sit waiting in the Pre-Operative Area—the causes are many and vary with the type of institution (i.e. University Teaching Hospital vs. Ambulatory Surgery Centre)

Your Time in the Operating Room — Your experience in the Operating Room will likely be that of a fast-paced environment where you are the centre of attention—many of the activities in preparing for surgery are under your influence and control; accepting that most of the activities that occur within the Operating Room are outside your control will be an important factor in letting go and reducing your anxiety

Your Vital Signs — Monitoring your vital signs is a tremendously important aspect of your anesthesia and surgical care—refer to Appendix C for a description of the various monitors that you'll encounter in the Operating Room

A Checklist to Keep You Safe — The Surgical Safety Checklist is another tool developed by the WHO to optimize communication and keep you safe in the Operating Room—ask your institution if they use a checklist in their Operating Rooms

An Anesthetic That's Right for You — Your anesthetic can take many forms and include the categories of general anesthesia (going to sleep), regional anesthesia (a large part of your body is numb) and local anesthesia (a small, specific part of your body is numb)—sedation is common with regional and local anesthetics (see Chapter 3 for details)

Your IV — If you've had difficulties getting an intravenous (IV) catheter in the past or have small, difficult-to-see veins, see the Insider Tip "Making the IV Easier on You"

Your Recovery from Anesthesia — The Post-Anesthetic Care Unit is where you'll typically recover from your anesthetic—from here, you'll be prepared to move on to either the Hospital Ward or through the process of being discharged

Managing Your Recovery from Anesthesia — Common issues following surgery include a sore throat, nausea and vomiting, poor short-term memory and pain—you'll have a team in the Post-Anesthetic Care Unit dedicated to identifying and treating these issues; be sure to communicate your symptoms as best you can to help the team tailor treatment to meet your needs

Your Memory After Anesthesia — Poor short-term memory immediately after anesthesia is very common and a cause of many instructions and details about the surgery being forgotten by the patient—if post-operative instructions aren't provided in writing, ask for a loved one to be present when important pieces of information are being shared at this time

Communicating Your Pain — Proper pain control is important when recovering from surgery—rate your pain on a scale of 0 to 10 (0 = no pain; 10 = excruciating pain) for your team so they can work to keep your pain well controlled; you must be able to breathe deeply and move as expected to keep your early recovery on track

Key Takeaway from Chapter 3

- Your active participation throughout the day of surgery is vital for optimal communication, risk reduction and optimizing your early recovery

Chapter 4 Summary—Recovery from Surgery

Essential Information

Your Recovery Time — The time it will take for you to recover from surgery will likely be much longer than the operation itself

Your Recovery Location — Your recovery will occur in one or more of the following locations: 1) Hospital Ward; 2) Intensive Care Unit; 3) Home—an abbreviated list of considerations for each location is included below

Your Recovery in Hospital
- Your work with healthcare professionals should be on level ground—they are experts in clinical care; you are the expert on you—expect collaboration

- You'll work with numerous professionals if you spend time recovering on the Hospital Ward—the better you understand their roles, the more effectively and accurately you can share your needs and discuss the plan for your care (find descriptions for many of these professionals in Chapter 4)

- Knowing the plan—understanding the plan for your care, knowing what is expected of you, sharing your concerns and what is important to you are among the best ways to make sure your recovery stays on track

- Deep breathing, appropriate movement/exercise, proper nutrition and looking after your skin and wound(s) are all vital elements of your recovery—together, addressing these elements have the ability to reduce the length of your stay in hospital, prevent re-admission to hospital and reduce your risk of complications (if part of your recovery will be on the Hospital Ward, I encourage you to read the section in Chapter 4 called "Your Job on the Ward")

Your Medications & Pain Control

- While you should expect some pain after surgery, the goal is to reduce your discomfort so that it is mild and quite tolerable

- Be honest when rating your pain and realize that pain is subjective and everyone experiences it differently—this highlights the value of using a rating scale to communicate this (e.g. 0 = no pain; 10 = excruciating pain)

- Be proactive in treating your pain—pain medications don't work immediately so don't wait for pain to be too intense before taking the prescribed dose

- Deep breathing and doing your prescribed exercises are vital to a good recovery—if pain is preventing this, be sure to work with your healthcare team to optimize your pain control

- All medications have potential side effects and some can cause allergic reactions—report side effects to your doctor and consider allergic reactions a medical emergency worthy of a visit to an Emergency Room

- 5 Questions—read the one-page reference in Chapter 4 called "5 Questions to Ask About Your Medications"—this applies to anyone taking medications for any reason

Your Tests After Surgery

- Visit choosingwiselycanada.org (or choosingwisely.org if you live in the US) to learn about having discussions and making informed decisions about medical tests—it's important to avoid unnecessary tests, treatments and procedures

Infection Prevention & Control

- Infections of your surgical wound are the most common type of infection after surgery

- To reduce your risk, do the following: 1) Wash your hands; 2) Ensure your care providers wash their hands; 3) Ask visitors to wash their hands; 4) If you have diabetes, control your blood sugar; 5) If you smoke, do your best to quit or reduce smoking as much as possible

Your Recovery in the Intensive Care Unit
- An Intensive Care Unit (ICU) is a specialty department within a hospital designed to care for patients who require continuous monitoring and active treatment of conditions that pose an immediate threat to their health
- You may need to recover in an ICU if you have a serious pre-existing medical condition, complex surgery, emergency surgery or complications during surgery

Your Recovery at Home
- Once you leave for home, you are leaving many healthcare professionals behind, along with their answers to your questions and their timely directions—this is fine as long as you prepare well before you leave
- Use your Ready for My Surgery Checklist to guide your questions and write down important instructions and information—don't rely on your memory
- Arrange for a loved one to take you home and stay with you for the minimum amount of time recommended to you
- Recovering from surgery can be hard—stay focused on restoring yourself to good health, the best that is possible for your situation
- Consider this time to be an opportunity to take full control over your health—create new routines around exercise, nutrition and rest

Key Takeaway from Chapter 4

- Be it at hospital or home, the success of your recovery is influenced directly by your diligence in understanding the plan for your recovery, communicating your needs and fulfilling your role

Chapter 5 Summary—Giving Feedback & Giving Back

Essential Information

Your Perspective   Your perspective as a patient is unique—consider sharing your experience and insights to support the continuous improvement of your healthcare system

Your Voice — Visit www.readyformysurgery.com/survey to share what you've learned and have your voice heard—you could create a better experience for those who follow you

Your Feedback — Take full advantage of opportunities to give both positive and constructive feedback to your hospital and the care providers you worked with—be specific, be constructive, do it as soon as possible and focus on things that can be changed

Your Support — Would you enjoy being actively involved with your local healthcare institution? There are many ways to give back—volunteering your time, offering your financial support, sharing your expertise—such contributions help hospitals achieve many important goals

Key Takeaway from Chapter 5

- Giving your perspective, feedback, time, expertise or money are all great ways to participate in the growth of your local healthcare institution

You have the power to influence the outcome of your surgery. Don't underestimate just how important this could be. To learn more, continue on to Chapter 1.

1

SCHEDULED FOR SURGERY

PURPOSE OF THIS CHAPTER
To offer key insights into the reality of having surgery and first steps for you to take.

KEY THINGS WE'LL COVER
- Why it's important for you to be informed and engaged
- *Yikes!* Thoughts and emotions about surgery
- What *you* can do to influence your outcome
- A little about medical tests and appointments

GREAT... SURGERY.

Perhaps you're looking forward to having a needed surgery. Or, perhaps not... Regardless, a wide range of emotions can accompany the anticipation of an operation. In my experience, even the most stoic of people experience some anxiety. Sometimes, it doesn't hit until you're lying on the Operating Room table.

Hey, the nerves can get to any of us! I can clearly recall one patient who was both laughing and crying as she lay on the OR table—really, she was laughing at herself for crying. A flood of emotion. We talked and laughed with her, reassuring her that we go through many boxes of tissues for such occasions. She was not alone—this was our message—not alone in her experience of feeling scared, nor alone during her surgery. Our common goal at that moment was to care for her as a person, not just a patient. This is where the compassion of healthcare professionals makes the biggest (and longest-lasting) impact on their patients.

Reassuring? Maybe not.

However, if you are feeling a little uneasy about surgery, it can be helpful to explore some of the reasons for this apprehension. The mind is a wonderful thing but it can wander—and wandering around the topic of surgery without many facts (beyond a few tidbits from *Grey's Anatomy*) can lead to scary places! As you read on, we'll explore the facts about this journey (along with some interesting stories), beginning with some first steps and things to consider now that you're scheduled for surgery.

Why Should I Bother Reading About All This?

"I don't want to know anything... let's just get this over with!"

If I had a nickel...

There have been no shortage of patients who offered some variation of this statement to me over the years. Who could blame them? It's not such a fun topic—the surgery was happening to *them*, after all.

Consider this: The surgery itself is actually just one part of the entire journey you'll embark upon. An important part, yes, but just one part. Your preparation before the day of surgery can impact your outcome, for better or for worse depending on what you do. Your participation on the day of surgery is also vital. Every patient has a role to play and should expect to participate in their healthcare. Important decisions about your care will happen—ensure you have a seat at the table when they do.

No one cares about the outcome of your surgery as much as you do—not the doctors, not the nurses—you're the one who will live with the final result.

Don't leave it to chance. You can't control everything, but you can control your part.

Something else to think about: The time it will take to perform your operation will be short relative to the duration of your recovery. Knowing in advance what you can expect during your recovery will help you to plan accordingly, bring in the resources you need and find answers before you end up home with only questions and concerns.

That said, let's quickly get you the place where you are prepared for this journey ahead. To get started, we'll explore a few essential questions.

🔍 SHOW ME THE EVIDENCE

In healthcare, we're used to talking about **THE EVIDENCE**. Well, it turns out that understanding your role as a patient and being prepared to manage your health and healthcare has been linked to better health outcomes. (Yay, keep reading!) The topic of research that applies to us here is categorized by the terms "Patient Engagement" or "Patient Activation" (you'll know when you're activated... Shazam!). This research is diverse in terms of the types of healthcare scenarios being evaluated (e.g. chronic conditions, hospitalized patients, patient safety, healthcare utilization, and so on). It turns out that you're more likely to prepare questions related to your health, take better care of yourself, spend less time in hospital and have fewer adverse events when you're actively involved.[1,2]

---

[1] John Andrawis et al., "Higher Preoperative Patient Activation Associated with Better Patient-Reported Outcomes After Total Joint Arthroplasty." *Clinical Orthopaedics and Related Research* (2015), https://www.ncbi.nlm.nih.gov/pmc/articles/PMC4488208/.

[2] Jessica Greene et al., "When Patient Activation Levels Change, Health Outcomes and Costs Change, Too." *Health Affairs* (2015), https://www.healthaffairs.org/doi/full/10.1377/hlthaff.2014.0452.

Are My Feelings About Surgery Normal?

Yes—whatever those feelings may be. For many people having an operation, this will be the first time they have had any significant interaction with their healthcare system. Or maybe they've had previous interactions that weren't so pleasant.

Many will have never set foot inside a hospital. Others know the hospital all too well. Some people feel lost in these huge buildings with people rushing every which way.

When we're out of our element, treading through unfamiliar environments, a sense of unease may come our way in the form of:

- Anxiety
- Nervousness
- Feeling a lack of control
- Frustration
- Fear
- Anger
- Sadness
- Curiosity
- Confusion

> **INSIDER TIP**
>
> A little side note about feeling lost—the truth is, many of the people working in the hospital get lost in there too! Maybe I'm a slow learner, but it took me months before I knew all the back staircases, shortcuts and how the floors of hospital wing 1 matched up with hospital wings 2 & 3 that were built 20–30 years later and had been mashed together. So, don't be overly surprised when you ask for directions and the person in scrubs looks as confused as you do. Through my helpful efforts, I undoubtedly pointed many a patient in the wrong direction... Sorry! Now, back to feelings.

These are the emotions that patients present to healthcare professionals every day. By dealing with these now, you'll free yourself up to focus on the actions you can take to give yourself the best chance for success.

Everyone will manage their thoughts and emotions uniquely, however, here are a couple points to consider if you're struggling a little:

GRATITUDE

Access to high-quality healthcare is a privilege. Many do not have this luxury. Having the opportunity for your health to be looked after by experts with an arsenal of medical and surgical options is something to be thankful for.

ACCEPTANCE

Focus on the things you can control and accept those you cannot. In this book, we're going to focus on the things you can control. By helping you become a truly informed and engaged patient, you will be much better prepared to accept the elements of care that you cannot directly control.

WHAT OPPORTUNITY DOES THIS PRESENT?

It is not a new thought to suggest that with challenges come opportunities, but it is a powerful one. Perhaps this surgery is the wake-up call you needed to start eating better, begin an exercise program or convince you to quit smoking once and for all. It may be the trigger that invites you to slow down and reflect on the things that matter most, to think about where you spend your time and energy.

What does this make possible? Discover the opportunity.

How Can You Influence the Care You Receive?

Be an informed healthcare consumer. This means that you pay attention to the state of your health, you ask questions about your care and you reflect upon and share what is important to you. There is enormous benefit to being informed. As we move through the various stages of the journey to and from the hospital, the benefits will become apparent.

Where Do I Start?

For you, this depends on when you get to this page in the book. Maybe you've already discussed your need for surgery with your family doctor (also commonly referred to as a primary care physician or general practitioner). If not, you should. They will know your medical history well and will use this knowledge to give you information and advice about your surgery.

Family doctors play a very important role in ensuring that you are fit for surgery and can order tests related to areas of concern. These tests can include blood work, x-rays, CT scans, MRIs and ECGs (we'll cover these a little later). Your surgeon could order these too.

Be sure to get these tests out of the way to ensure your surgery isn't delayed. Meet with your family doctor after surgery too. Schedule follow-up appointments now—when you're not preoccupied recovering from your operation.

📣 CALL TO ACTION

What is your single biggest fear, concern or challenge related to your surgery? Think it over then write it down (I'll give you a good spot to do this shortly). Talk about it with others—your family, friends, healthcare providers, whomever you think could help you address it. Wouldn't it be great if you could reduce the impact this has on you?

If you don't have a family doctor, consider trying to find one. There are organizations that regulate the practice of medicine in different regions; these are called *Regulatory Colleges*. In Canada, each province has a Regulatory College for physicians which offer ways to search for a family doctor. Here are two examples:

Ontario: www.cpso.on.ca/Public-Information-Services/Find-a-Doctor
Alberta: search.cpsa.ca/physiciansearch
For a Canada-wide listing of physician regulatory colleges, visit fmrac.ca/members/.

Other countries may have similar resources. If you live in the United States, the American Medical Association has a search tool called DoctorFinder that you can access here: doctorfinder.ama-assn.org/doctorfinder/home.jsp.

What Should I Know About My Health?

Like any other part of your life, such as your finances or career, understanding your health issues and how to manage them reduces the risk of unexpected consequences. For example, blindly handing over your hard-earned money to a near-stranger at your local financial institution may work out okay, but what control do you have over the outcome? You know your financial goals best and by being financially literate, you can help ensure your plan stays on track, which can reduce your risk of being surprised with the results.

Much the same, many people place their faith solely in the healthcare providers they encounter and invest very little into understanding their health, their role as a patient and the basics of their healthcare. Congratulations to you for making that investment. The benefits are significant and even have the potential to improve the outcome of your surgical journey.

What If I Have an Underlying Illness?

Do you have a chronic (long-term) health issue? If so, you're not alone. In fact, the majority of people scheduled for an operation have some type of issue with their health. Rest assured that the team of healthcare professionals you'll meet at the hospital is quite accustomed to this and will be very interested in hearing about your health history.

Interviewing patients prior to surgery was part of my daily routine as a clinician. It sometimes took a lot of digging—more like detective work, really—to uncover the full health history (we hoped) of some patients. And while I enjoy a good mystery as much as the next person, let's not have the story of *your* health be one filled with shadowy places, twists and turns. By the end of this book, you'll have the tools to ensure your story will be clear, concise and complete. The benefit will be that the management of your medical care can likewise be clear and focused.

Prior to your surgery, a major focus will be to ensure that any chronic illnesses you have are kept as stable as possible. Here are some of the most common conditions:

- High blood pressure
- Diabetes
- Obesity
- Chronic obstructive pulmonary disease (COPD)
- Heart disease
- Asthma
- Obstructive sleep apnea

While we won't be exploring these health issues in detail in this book, it's important that you understand your health issues, the impact they have on your well-being, how to manage them and how to know that your condition is stable.

Enhanced Recovery After Surgery

Sounds like something I'd want!

An organization called the ERAS Society (ERAS stands for Enhanced Recovery After Surgery—erassociety.org/patients) has developed guidelines that have been shown to improve how quickly you recover after an operation. It turns out that there are some simple things you can do that can help you recover more quickly, have fewer complications and leave the hospital sooner.

Not all hospitals use ERAS protocols but it's becoming more common because of the strong evidence to support them. At the time of the writing of this book, a pan-Canadian initiative called Enhanced Recovery Canada is just beginning. Over twenty organizations across Canada have begun working together to increase the awareness and use of ERAS protocols in Canadian hospitals. This work is being led by the Canadian Patient Safety Institute (CPSI) and they'd be thrilled if you visited their website to see how this project is progressing (www.patientsafety institute.ca). In the US, two great places to learn about ERAS-related work include the ERAS Society USA Chapter (erasusa.org) and the American Society for Enhanced Recovery (aserhq.org).

Here's a snapshot of some common elements of an ERAS protocol. Take note that your particular protocol may vary based on your surgery, your health and your hospital.

BEFORE SURGERY	DURING SURGERY	AFTER SURGERY
↓	↓	↓
Exercise, healthy diet, stop smoking	Smaller incisions, less IV fluids	Out of bed often and as soon as possible
↓	↓	↓
Pre-operative visit to discuss your care plan	Pain control using spinals, epidurals and nerve blocks	Eating and drinking as soon as possible
↓	↓	↓
Eating usually until 8 hours before surgery	Less morphine and other similar drugs	Preventative control of nausea and vomiting
↓	↓	↓
Drinking clear fluids until 2 hours before	Strategies to reduce nausea and vomiting	Less IV fluids and less morphine and similar drugs

Nutrition & Surgery

Let's talk a little more about proper eating before surgery. The focus on optimizing a person's nutritional state before surgery is likely to become more of a focus in the future. Why? There is evidence that suggests that if you are malnourished going into surgery, you're more likely to have a complication afterward and are more likely to be re-admitted to the hospital.[3]

A Registered Dietician is well prepared to help you determine this, although only a minority of patients get a nutritional consult before an operation. The big question for you is if *you* need a boost in your nutrition before you head in for surgery.

Is your nutrition good enough for surgery?

Registered Dieticians and Naturopathic Doctors are skilled and focused on nutrition. They can best assess your current status and give recommendations before and after surgery. Here are a few scenarios that should lead you to consider meeting with a nutrition specialist before surgery:[4]

---

3 American College of Surgeons, "Optimizing Nutrition Prior to Surgery," https://www.facs.org/quality-programs/strong-for-surgery/clinicians/nutrition.

4 Paul E. Wischmeyer et al., "American Society for Enhanced Recovery and Perioperative Quality Initiative Joint Consensus Statement on Nutrition Screening and Therapy Within a Surgical Enhanced Recovery Pathway." *Anesthesia and Analgesia* (2018), https://www.ncbi.nlm.nih.gov/pubmed/29369092.

- You've lost weight recently
- Your Body Mass Index (BMI) is less than 18.5 kg/m² (if your age is less than 20 or above 65)
- You've been eating a lot less than usual
- You take steroids for a medical condition
- Your immune system is suppressed (due to medication or a condition, such as cancer)
- You are having surgery on your esophagus, stomach or colon

Remember to stay hydrated up until the deadline you were given; you should generally be able to drink water or clear juice up until two hours before your surgery. Confirm that you can do this with your surgeon or anesthesiologist, and then drink up.

Smoking & Surgery

There is one topic that deserves exploring a little further here—smoking. If you don't smoke, feel free to skip over this section. If you do smoke, hang in with me on this... just for a short time. There are a few pretty good reasons not to blow me off just yet.

My dad has smoked since he was a teenager. He tried to quit a bunch of times over the years. He even managed to quit for an extended period a couple of times. Unfortunately, it didn't last. The truth was, as my dad would later tell me, he didn't really want to quit.

Sound familiar? I get it.

On the other hand, I'm trained as a Respiratory Therapist. As such, an innate desire to keep your lungs healthy has been ingrained into my subconscious. My goal with this book is simply to help you make informed decisions—this topic is no different. Please have a read through this Insider Tip and see what you think. Later on in the book, we'll talk about the hard parts of having surgery—this just might be the hardest part for you, but that doesn't mean you shouldn't face it.

💡 INSIDER TIP

SMOKING & SURGERY

THE CHALLENGE

Globally, about 1 in 5 people over 15 years of age smoke tobacco.

In some countries, half the men are smokers. Unfortunately, adolescents have high rates of smoking too, spurred largely from targeted advertising by the tobacco industry.

Do you smoke?

Have you ever tried to quit? If you have and were successful, congratulations.

Have you tried to quit without success? If so, don't be hard on yourself—nicotine (the addictive substance in tobacco) is just as addictive as cocaine and heroin.

Maybe you'd like to quit but have been waiting for the right time. Well, you're in luck.

THE FACTS

Now don't worry—there'll be no lecturing here, we're just going to cover the facts. To be clear though, my goal is to help you stop smoking before surgery (and hopefully for good). Since research shows that 70% of smokers want to quit, the odds are that you are one of them.[5] As you'll see, this is really a great opportunity for you to make this change.

You already know that smoking isn't good for your lungs. That's not all, though; it negatively affects your heart function, blood circulation and more.

Let's not focus on the usual bad stuff though... you've probably heard enough of that. Let's focus on the big wins you can achieve with small steps:

12 HOURS—let's start with that—what benefits could possibly exist after quitting smoking for such a short time?

Your body is amazing—after only 12 hours after quitting your body begins to heal and your heart, lungs and blood circulation start to improve! The benefits of this to you are:[6]

- Faster healing of your surgical wound
- Less risk of infection
- Less risk of coughing after surgery (this places unwanted strain on some incisions)
- Less risk of getting pneumonia
- Less risk of having a heart attack
- Less risk of needing a ventilator to support your breathing after surgery

These are kind of a big deal, right?! The longer you quit before surgery, the greater ability your body has to manage these risks. It's not clear exactly how early you need to quit to have the greatest benefit but the sooner the better is fair to say. To be a little more precise, think weeks rather than days.

It's also worth noting that you can't smoke in the hospital. As a result, some smokers experience nicotine withdrawal during their in-hospital recovery. As you can imagine, adding withdrawal symptoms to the challenge of recovering from surgery is an experience worth avoiding.

THE OPPORTUNITY

The big opportunity is this: If you stop smoking before surgery, you've taken an important first step down the path to quitting altogether. You'll have days or even weeks free of smoking by the time of your operation.

During the time you're in the hospital, you'll not be able to smoke either (more days added to kicking the habit). By the

---

5 Stephen Babb et al., "Quitting Smoking Among Adults—United States, 2000–2015." *Morbidity and Mortality Weekly Report* (2017), http://dx.doi.org/10.15585/mmwr.mm6552a1.

6 American Society of Anesthesiologists, "When Seconds Count—Risks—Smoking," https://www.asahq.org/whensecondscount/preparing-for-surgery/risks/smoking/.

time you go home, you'll have made some tremendous steps toward quitting smoking for good!

Studies show that a large percentage of people who quit smoking before surgery will be non-smokers a year later. If you can do this, here are the added benefits:

- You'll could add a good 6–10 years to your life, depending on the age you quit[7] (just think about that)
- You'll avoid exposing your family and friends to harmful secondhand smoke
- You'll have more cash in your pocket—potentially over a thousand dollars a year
- You'll reduce your risk of getting awful diseases, such as lung cancer, heart disease and stroke[8] (don't underestimate just how awful these are)

Consider your surgery an opportunity to make this important change. The fact that you've made it this far into this book means that you're committed to achieving a positive outcome for your operation—if you're a smoker, one of the most important things you can do to this end is quit smoking before surgery.

You can do it. And you should.

DON'T TRY TO DO IT ALONE
Why not? Because it's hard. And hard things are more easily accomplished with help. There are tools and experts that can help you. Nicotine patches alone double your odds of quitting. Expert counsellors have done all the research for you. They've coached many people to successfully stop smoking.

Are you resisting this idea of getting help? Some people do—that's okay. Humour me for a moment and think about the last time you asked someone for assistance—the hardware store, the Apple Store... Why did you ask? Because you knew that they had the expertise and knowledge that could help you achieve your goal. Be it buying the right light bulb or laptop computer, talking to experts helps us make good decisions and avoid mistakes.

The thing is, you may need more than a nicotine patch to help you quit. Your odds of success increase as you add counselling and other interventions to the mix. Everyone is different and what works for one person may not do the trick for another. Speaking with an expert on smoking cessation (preferably, more than once) allows for a personalized plan to be put into place for you. If you really want this, get an expert on your side.

WHERE TO FIND HELP
In Canada, the Canadian Cancer Society's Smokers' Helpline offers free counselling. To access this service, visit www.smokershelpline.ca or call 1-877-513-5333.

In the United States, a national counselling service is available to anyone wanting to quit smoking at 1-800-QUIT-NOW.

---

7 Prabhat Jha et al., "21st-Century Hazards of Smoking and Benefits of Cessation in the United States." *New England Journal of Medicine* (2013), https://www.nejm.org/doi/10.1056/NEJMsa1211128.

8 US Department of Health and Human Services, "Surgeon General's Report on Smoking and Health: 1964–2014," https://www.hhs.gov/sites/default/files/consequences-smoking-consumer-guide.pdf.

If you're a young adult, this resource was made for you: leavethepackbehind.org.

No matter where you live, check out www.stopsmokingforsafersurgery.ca. You'll hear from a Canadian anesthesiologist about his experience giving anesthetics to smokers. As you'll read, the issues related to smoking and surgery aren't just theoretical. I like this resource because it began as a personal effort to make a difference. That's cool.

Take this opportunity and get it done. Good luck.

PLEASE LET ME KNOW

If you took your surgery as the opportunity to quit smoking, I'd love to know! Email me at patrick.nellis@readyformysurgery.com—you could be an inspiration for others. These are the important stories to tell.

Talking to Others

It can be reassuring to talk about your upcoming surgery, not just with your doctor but also with friends and family. It isn't difficult to find someone who has spent time in hospital for a procedure. The unknown can be a source of anxiety, so why not talk to someone who has been through it? Not everyone has a cheerful story about their surgery—it is surgery after all. However, hearing a personal story of their journey will give you a better idea of what to expect. Seek out people who have your best interests in mind and won't take this as an opportunity to simply indulge in their own story.

A Chance Conversation

While writing this book, I happened to chat with an acquaintance I'd made doing some community volunteer work. Football had taken its toll on Bill's knees in his younger days—now he was in line for a knee replacement. He mentioned it to me one day and we ended up talking about it.

It was pretty clear that no one had given him a good breakdown of how this knee replacement would actually go down. We talked for a while and since I'd been in the OR for hundreds of hip and knee replacements, I was able to walk him through what to expect.

I didn't see Bill for a while after his surgery. He was home, diligently doing his physiotherapy and healing up (we'd talked about the consequences that await those who don't). The next time I saw him, he seemed almost amazed and surprised that his experience surrounding his surgery was just as I'd described. For you, dear reader, we'll take it one step further—informed and empowered is the goal.

Getting Help

Now is the time to ask for support. Think about people in your life that can help out, whether that be with a warm bowl of soup, a ride to and from the hospital or someone who can motivate you to stay active when you need it. Speak with your healthcare team if you need assistance finding necessary supports.

You'll want someone to take you to the hospital and bring you back home. Once you arrive home, you may need help for even simple activities of daily living, depending on your limitations after surgery. For example, you may have difficulty moving around and you may need to avoid certain activities for a period of time.

As well, many pain medications used after surgery have side effects that can impact your ability to look after yourself, let alone anyone else. Pain and pain medications will be discussed in Chapter 4.

A Tip for Moms & Dads

Hospitals can be scary and overwhelming for children. Be sure to include them in the process. Their age and understanding will determine how much you decide to tell them.

If they're old enough, let them know how *they* can help! Hospitals are special places. Have them visit the hospital with you if you can. If you'll remain as an in-patient after surgery, your kids will likely find visiting you there a lot easier if they have already done some exploring.

Getting Organized

Okay, there are going to be a lot of things for you to keep track of. To start, you'll need a list of all your medications (and dosages), appointment information, items to bring to the hospital, special instructions for the day of surgery, etc. And there's more, lots more...

Is it *really* that important to have your ducks in a row? Allow me to convince you that it is.

Not being able to accurately provide information about your health and the medications you take will prevent your healthcare providers from fully understanding your state of health. This has a *direct* impact on your surgery, anesthesia and pain management.

How? Let's say that I'm looking after your anesthetic and you're having a knee replacement (don't worry, it's just for illustration!). I'll want to have a very clear picture of your current state of health, any previous surgeries you've had and if you'd had any issues with those surgeries.

I'll ask a number of questions about your medications too. Not just *what* medications you take (including the over-the-counter ones) but also *how long* you've been taking them, the dose of those drugs and if that dose had been *changed recently* (this will give me a hint about the stability of the condition for which the drug was prescribed). As for drugs not sold in pharmacies (i.e. street drugs), you can share your habits in confidence. And you should. Recreational drugs such as marijuana, illicit opioids and alcohol can significantly affect how much anesthetic you require. In fact, a higher dose of anesthetic is often needed for people who regularly use these drugs. If anesthesia care providers are unaware of this, they are far more likely to underdose the anesthetic—not what you want! It's worth being honest about this, even if it is uncomfortable. I'll also ask you about allergies, family history and more—then I'll ask you if you have any questions or concerns.

Whoa.

Imagine trying to pull all that stuff out of your brain in the minutes just prior to going into the OR... Oh, and you'll not have had breakfast or your morning coffee to help you out either. It'll be kind of like going through a tough job interview and then being asked if you have any questions at the end. If you haven't prepared beforehand, it can be a challenge to answer the questions well and then also ask about the things that really matter to you.

Let's say you've had a reaction in the past to an antibiotic but forget to mention it in that moment. Maybe you're allergic to shellfish and don't offer this tidbit because you don't see how it could be relevant to your surgery. Or, you had nausea and vomiting after your last anesthetic and think of it only as you're experiencing the same after this one (a potentially preventable and problematic complication). Maybe your biggest fear is having pain after surgery but just before you were about to share this, they tell you that the OR is ready and you don't want to hold things up by asking questions (you don't want to be a bother, of course).

These are a few examples (there are dozens more) that highlight how easy it is to forget or omit key pieces of information on the day of surgery. All the information you provide is used to tailor your healthcare to meet *your* needs. You want things to go smoothly—you can eliminate risks by getting organized and understanding your health. Remember, you're part of your healthcare team. Do your part.

We'll get organized together to help make this road a little safer.

> ### 📣 CALL TO ACTION
>
> **INTRODUCING YOUR READY FOR MY SURGERY CHECKLIST**
>
> Time to flip to Appendix A. This is your tool to get organized. Each section of this checklist is clearly labelled and ready for you to add all the information you'll need before, during and after the day of your surgery. Everything's all in one place—easy for you to reference and easy to share with anyone that needs to know.
>
> There are 8 sections for you to complete:
>
> 1. My Hospital
> 2. My Surgery
> 3. My Surgeon
> 4. My Appointments
> 5. My Health
> 6. Day of Surgery
> 7. Other Things to Bring
> 8. My Recovery
>
> We'll not only have you organized but this checklist will also highlight for you what information is important. So, let's take the guesswork out of your preparation—pull out your Ready for My Surgery Checklist and pull in the people needed to get those boxes checked off! We'll keep working on this throughout the book.

Appointments Before Surgery

Just as you and I will be working to get things in order, your healthcare team will also be looking to do the same. Meeting with you and preparing in advance of your operation will ensure that everyone has all the information needed to set you up for a good outcome. You may be referred to a medical specialist if you have any medical conditions that need to be optimized. Such specialists include respirologists (lung doctors, also known as pulmonologists), cardiologists (heart doctors) and endocrinologists (hormone doctors, specializing in diseases such as diabetes). In this next section, we'll cover the Pre-Admission Clinic, followed by a short overview of some of the common medical tests you may need.

Pre-Admission Clinic

The better prepared you are, the quicker and easier your visit to the Pre-Admission Clinic will be. Here you'll have a medical assessment where much of the information gathering takes place (your prep work will pay off here).

Typically, an anesthesiologist and/or nurse will interview you. He or she will review your health history, ask you about your allergies and discuss with you how to manage your medications for the surgery. Issues and instructions related to the surgery and your anesthetic will also be reviewed, such as the likelihood of receiving a blood transfusion. While at the clinic you may also require blood tests, x-rays or other tests according to your situation. *A little side note here: Some patients are surprised on the day of surgery when their anesthesiologist is not the same person they met in the Pre-Admission Clinic. This is a fairly common occurrence since many patients are seen in the clinic on any given day. If this is the case for you, rest assured that your anesthesia care provider will have access to a report summarizing the information gathered during your Pre-Admission Clinic visit.*

Not every person is going to be scheduled for a pre-admission appointment. Your surgeon will decide that and the office will let you know if it is required. Sometimes, only a phone interview is needed if you are relatively healthy and the surgery is considered minor. If you are scheduled to be there in person, suffice it to say that it is important to go—mandatory to go. The information collected there will ensure the healthcare team is prepared for your surgery; missing the appointment may result in postponing or even cancelling your surgery.

> **INSIDER TIP**
>
> If you have been told that you have an antibiotic-resistant infection, such as MRSA, *C. difficile* or VRE, or if you have flu-like symptoms, call the clinic before your appointment for instructions. Why? These are the "super bugs" you may have heard about. They're tough to treat because many of the usual antibiotics don't work on them. These germs are particularly dangerous to hospital patients whom often have weakened immune systems.

Medical Tests

There are a variety of tests you may require ahead of your operation. Maybe you're already familiar with tests like x-rays, CT scans or MRIs. If not, or if you'd just like to learn a little more, feel free to skip to Appendix B where you'll find a brief description of the following tests:

- X-ray
- Computerized Tomography (CT) scan
- Magnetic Resonance Imaging (MRI)
- Ultrasound
- Endoscopy
- Electrocardiogram (ECG/EKG)
- Pulmonary Function Testing (PFT)
- Blood work

> ### 📣 CALL TO ACTION
> Write down the details of all your tests into the "My Appointments" section of your Ready for My Surgery Checklist. Easy, right?

Choose Wisely

I'd like to introduce you to a Canadian campaign called Choosing Wisely Canada designed to help you and your doctors discuss medical tests *before* they are ordered. As you'll see, conversations about unnecessary testing are relevant no matter where you live. Here's how they describe their work: "Choosing Wisely Canada is a campaign to help clinicians and patients engage in conversations about unnecessary tests, treatments and procedures" (choosingwiselycanada.org).

This organization has provided an exceptional resource to empower people to ask questions and make smart decisions about medical tests—everything from x-rays and CT scans to heart tests and even pain medications. As a foundation for these conversations, here are four questions they recommend that you ask your doctor about medical tests:

1. Do I really need this test, treatment or procedure?
1. What are the downsides?
2. Are there simpler, safer options?
3. What happens if I do nothing?

Take the time to visit choosingwiselycanada.org to learn more (or visit choosingwisely.org if you live in the US). Here's an example of some of the tests you'll be given guidance on (I picked the ones related to surgery for us):

Tests Before Surgery:
- Chest x-rays before surgery: When you need them—and when you don't
- Echocardiogram before surgery: When you need it—and when you don't
- Heart tests before surgery: When you need an imaging test—and when you don't
- Lab tests before surgery: When you need them—and when you don't

Check out the next page to see an example.

How great is that? By now, I'm sure you can appreciate just how many healthcare professionals and institutions are seeking to put you first—to bring you into the conversation as a partner in your healthcare. Join in.

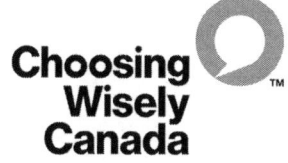

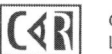 Canadian Association of Radiologists
L'Association canadienne des radiologistes

Choosing Wisely Canada is a campaign to help clinicians and patients engage in conversations about unnecessary tests and treatments and make smart and effective choices to ensure high-quality care.

For more information on Choosing Wisely Canada or to see other patient materials, visit choosingwiselycanada.org. Join the conversation on Twitter @ChooseWiselyCA

Chest X-rays before surgery
When you need them—and when you don't

Many people have a chest X-ray before they have surgery. This is called a "pre-op" chest X-ray. "Pre-op" stands for pre-operative, which means that it is before an operation, or surgery.

If you have a heart or lung disease, you may want to get a pre-op chest X-ray. It can show medical problems, like an enlarged heart, congestive heart failure, or fluid around the lungs. These could mean that your surgery should be delayed or cancelled. However, if you don't have signs or symptoms of a heart or lung disease, you should think twice about having a chest X-ray before surgery. Here's why:

A chest X-ray usually doesn't help.
Many people are given a chest X-ray to "clear" them before surgery. Some hospitals require a chest X-ray for almost every patient.

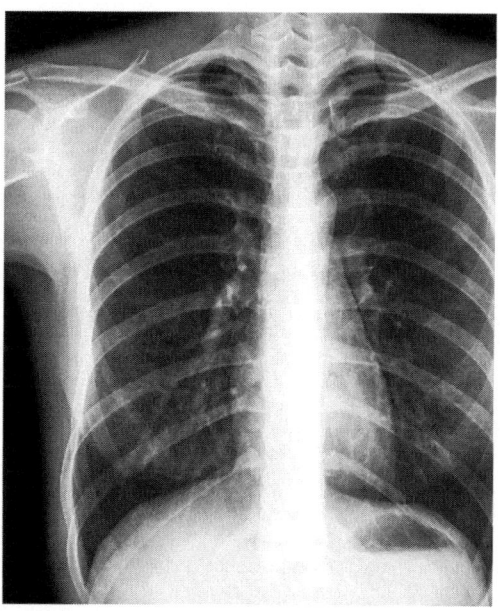

But, if you do not have symptoms of a heart or lung disease, and your risk is low, an X-ray probably will not help. It is not likely to show a serious problem that would change your treatment plan.

Choosing Wisely Canada (2017). Chest x-rays before surgery. Retrieved February 24, 2017 with permission from choosingwiselycanada.org

2

HOSPITALS & SURGERY CENTRES

PURPOSE OF THIS CHAPTER
To prevent surprises and reduce stress on the day of surgery by giving you some key tips to navigating the hospital.

KEY THINGS WE'LL COVER
- Types of places where surgery is performed (and why you should care to know)
- Getting there and getting around
- A quick introduction to healthcare providers

"TURN HERE."

"Which way?" said Steve.

"Left... no, right. And don't hit those people crossing the street!"

Mary hadn't been to this hospital before—had never cared to, in fact. She'd spent enough time in hospitals and doctors' offices when her mother was sick. It seems, though, that it was now her turn.

"*Look* at them. They're paying no attention... they just strut across the street like they own it," Steve muttered. He had a half a mind to give them a little nudge with his '09 Lucerne. He gave his head a shake instead.

He and Mary weren't big on the big city but this is where they were told they needed to be to get Mary's heart surgery looked after.

"There it is!" said Mary.

"Alright, now where the heck do we park?" Steve said. He was already a little fed up and they hadn't even set foot in the hospital yet.

GETTING THERE IS half the battle, they say. Steve and Mary aren't thrilled to be heading to the hospital—maybe you can relate? It can be stressful. There's a lot to prepare and think about. Having seen many patients appear frantic as they arrive for their operation, I can tell you that it's not the best way to start.

A little planning and organization will help you avoid a rough start to your day. Where to begin? Let's take quick peek inside the places that offer surgical services, then we'll talk about planning your trip.

> **💡 INSIDER TIP**
>
> The hallmarks of a University Teaching Hospital include leading-edge technologies, health research and advanced clinical care. As a patient here, you will have access to the most comprehensive healthcare, more specialists, larger teams and surgical techniques that aren't available elsewhere. If you have a health condition that is severe and potentially life-threatening, you may wish to discuss with your healthcare providers if a university hospital would be the best place for your surgery.

So, what type of hospital will you be visiting? Does it matter?

It could (otherwise, I wouldn't be bringing it up, I suppose). The way I look at it, it's all about what resources are available to you as a patient and the experience you can anticipate having. Think about your situation—*your* health—as you read through this next section and what your needs are.

University Teaching Hospitals, Community Hospitals and Surgery Centres all have notable differences, despite surgery as a common element. Many of these differences will influence your experience as a patient. All have unique advantages and limitations. Here's a quick overview that can help you understand what to expect from each.

University Teaching Hospitals

These hospitals are affiliated with medical schools and provide education and training to medical students, nurses, respiratory therapists, physiotherapists and other healthcare professionals. Generally, the most complex specialty surgeries and medical treatments are performed here, as well as research into new therapies and best practices.

What You Can Expect

- You are very likely to encounter students during a stay in a teaching hospital as a patient or visitor—this is good! I spent many years mentoring students at a teaching hospital. It is vital for learners to have supervised interactions with patients and visitors to help develop their clinical and interpersonal skills. Just as important, this interaction will also allow them to learn how crucial it is to include patients and their families in decision-making around their healthcare. Working together with patients so they can be informed and engaged in their healthcare is an important value to instill in all healthcare students. If you find yourself working with a student, don't be surprised if you find that you are asked to repeat some or all of what you said to the student's supervisor. This is to ensure your situation is properly understood and nothing has been missed.

- Teaching hospitals are typically large and difficult to navigate. Your planning will really pay off if this type of hospital is your destination.

- Emergency surgeries occur more commonly at teaching hospitals than anywhere else. This relates to the nature of their specialization and 24/7 availability of surgical services. A potential impact of an emergency surgery is the cancellation of elective (pre-booked) surgeries, *including yours*... This is a scenario I've seen many times. We'll talk more about this a little later.

Community Hospitals

These are the hospitals that serve most smaller and rural communities. While not all have a direct affiliation with a university, many healthcare students nonetheless receive valuable education here. They are focused on quality of patient care, efficiency and connecting with their community. These hospitals generally provide short-term medical care, routine surgical care and Emergency Room services.

What You Can Expect

- Often a warm, friendly reception. Small Community Hospitals tend to have staff that have worked together for many years. I've witnessed a closeness amongst staff at these hospitals that creates a relaxed, caring environment for patients.

- A desire for your support. Many Community Hospitals progress largely due to the involvement and generosity of members of their community. Significant interaction between the hospital and their community is facilitated by the Hospital Foundation. This is the hospital department that raises money for the hospital to help support its priorities for growth and development.

- High standards for patient care but fewer specialty services than University Teaching Hospitals. While Community Hospitals have highly skilled and knowledgeable staff, there will be situations in which the resources at a Community Hospital can no longer meet the needs of a few certain patients. In these cases, patients would then be transferred to a centre that has the resources to continue their care (yes, usually a university hospital). In reality, this point ends up applying to the minority of patients.

Ambulatory Surgery Centres (ASC)

If the surgery you're having is common and allows you to go home the same day, an ASC may be a great fit. These are also called same-day, or outpatient Surgery Centres. Only within the last few decades have ASCs become an option.

Ambulatory Surgery Centres focus on select types of procedures, such as ophthalmology (e.g. cataract surgery), endoscopy (e.g. colonoscopy) and chronic pain management. You are not likely to find other types of typical hospital services at these facilities, such as Emergency Room services. However, sometimes a Surgery Centre will be part of a multi-service health facility where you can have your x-rays, blood work, physiotherapy and follow-up appointments all in the same place. Pretty convenient. Arguably, very cost effective for the healthcare system too.

What You Can Expect

- Efficiency and specialization. These facilities thrive on their ability to refine and streamline the process of moving patients through every aspect of their surgery, from admission to discharge.

- Things can move fast here so be ready! I've supported hundreds of people during eye surgery as part of an Anesthesia Team at a specialized cataract clinic. This experience provided great insight into the efficiency potential of healthcare delivery.

- A positive experience. With such refined processes, the patient experience is often quite positive. Overall, ASCs have been shown to reduce the cost of procedures, take less time and can improve access to certain surgeries by reducing wait times.

- Greater limits when it comes to managing medical conditions. ASCs are great at what they do but if you have a serious medical condition, it is possible that your surgery will be scheduled at a hospital instead. This will allow for a longer monitoring period after surgery and access to more medical services if needed. Patients receiving care at an ASC may also be transferred to a hospital in the case of a medical emergency or an unstable medical condition.

📣 CALL TO ACTION

Find out what type of facility you'll be visiting for your surgery. Then, consider your health and the type of surgery you're having. Along with the information we just covered, ask yourself if it all fits. If it does, great. If something doesn't seem right, ask questions. Ask again, if you're not okay with the first answer. Persist if you need to—I've got your back.

Finding Your Way

Plan ahead; you'll be glad you did.

Give your appointment for surgery the attention it deserves and figure out the practical details, including travel, timing and stuff to bring. Most of your planning will be made easy by using your Ready for My Surgery Checklist—if you haven't yet, pull it out now and fill it in as we go along. To help us get started, here are some important questions to consider:

Where Am I Going?

Let's get some of the basic information down on paper. Start by writing down details about your hospital in your Ready for My Surgery Checklist (e.g. address, phone number, etc.). It sounds simple but it can be a help if you get lost along the way, you're running late or can't find the proper entrance—don't laugh, some hospitals are huge and have multiple entrances. All this information is available on the hospital's website (part of your checklist includes a spot to check off that you actually looked at it!). Hospital staff and volunteers are available to help you with directions and other information over the phone so give them a call if you'd like a little help.

Plan your mode of transportation and the route you'll take to the hospital ahead of time. You may feel a little anxious on the morning of the surgery and probably the night before too—having everything ready will keep things like planning your travel from adding to it.

Good Old Google
Planning alternate routes to the hospital in case of a traffic accident or unexpected road closure is pretty easy these days. If you haven't before, try Google Maps—just type it into any web browser on your computer or download the Google Maps mobile app on your smartphone or tablet. If you have a GPS in your car, that's great too.

When Do I Need to Arrive? (Don't Be Late!)

Once your surgery is booked, you'll be given a time to register at the hospital. Usually, it's a couple hours before your operation. Plan to be *early*. There's no need to add more stress to your day by rushing—or being late and having your surgery cancelled altogether… Write this information in your checklist (now's as good a time as any).

How Will I Get There?

Taxi or public transit are great ways to get to the hospital, especially since there will be no need for you to find or pay for parking. If you are driving, you'll have already wisely planned an alternate route to keep you on track.

Having someone else drive you is an even better idea. You could find yourself a little distracted on the morning of your surgery which isn't a great asset when it comes to driving. Ask a friend or family member to drive you (and pick you up) and work out the route and pick-up time between the two of you.

If I Decide to Drive, Where Is the Best Place to Park?

Beware of parking rates at hospitals! It can be extremely expensive to park at some hospitals, especially those located in large cities. Don't find yourself shocked at a huge parking fee following a hospital stay. Call the hospital ahead of time to find out their rates. With a little planning, you may save yourself a lot of money.

If you'll need parking for multiple days, most hospitals have weekly and monthly rates that will offer savings over daily rates. Explore other parking options—public lots can be cheaper.

What Do I Need to Bring?

The goal here is to bring what you need, nothing more. Travel light and have your things organized. During your surgery, you'll want to leave your valuables, including your wallet or purse, with your loved ones. Other items, such as clothes, will generally be placed in a bag labelled for you.

There is a section for this in your Ready for My Surgery Checklist. There you'll find a list of items to consider bringing to the hospital. This should prompt you to think carefully about the things you'll need and want during your hospital stay. Add to the list as you'd like.

For example, you should bring your dentures, hearing aids and glasses if you normally rely on them. If needed, these can often be used in the Operating Room until it's time for the anesthetic to be given. Your OR team will look after these items and ensure they are available when you need them again.

How Will I Get Home?

Generally, you'll need to have someone take you home after surgery. For many reasons, you won't be fit to get home by yourself.

If you're going home the same day as your surgery and you've received sedation medications or general anesthesia, these drugs will impair your ability to safely drive a vehicle. In this situation, you'll also need to avoid making any important decisions for the rest of that day (for example, don't plan to sell your house that night...).

If you've spent one or more nights in hospital, you may have had a more significant surgery and may be taking strong pain medications. On the day you go home, you may be faced with some challenges. Moving around may be an issue. You may also just feel like, well... like you've just had surgery. Your body is healing and is spending a lot of energy to do so. Take it easy. Enjoy the ride home from someone else.

Being Unprepared (Let's Actively Avoid This One)

I've seen many people arrive late for a scheduled surgery, or not at all. You can imagine the usual scenarios—slept in, traffic issues, forgot about it entirely... It's also not uncommon to have someone arrive to the hospital for major surgery after just eating a big, greasy breakfast (this happens to be a good way to get your surgery cancelled!). Some people won't have taken the medications they should have and some take the ones that were important not to take.

Being organized and informed is key to prevent all this. Carefully review the information provided to you by the surgeon's office when your appointment is scheduled. Use your Ready for My Surgery Checklist. This will help avoid preventable problems.

> **INSIDER TIP**
>
> Just don't forget your surgery appointment. Seriously? Oh, it happens. Imagine that you did... you'd feel awful—guilty and stressed. You'd have inconvenienced many people, including your surgeon and the OR team, other patients (that could have taken your place), the hospital (by wasting valuable OR time), your friends and family that had planned to help you, and yourself—you've now delayed your surgery, maybe complicated things at work, etc. Just don't forget—being organized and bringing in friends and family to help you out will minimize this risk.

CALL TO ACTION

Keep going on your Ready for My Surgery Checklist. Highlight the parts you can't answer and ask for help. Think about who knows you best—your family doctor, pharmacist, specialist, naturopathic doctor, family member, etc. Now's the time to get the details you need.

People You May Meet

Okay, I've asked you to do a lot of thinking just now—time for a break. In case you're not familiar with the variety of healthcare providers you may be working with in the hospital, let's briefly introduce them to you.

As you can imagine, all the activities surrounding your surgery require a team of professionals and support staff. Below is a high-level overview—we'll cover a little more about these folks later on when we discuss the specific role they play before, during and after your surgery.

Medical Doctors

"Hi, I'm Dr. So-and-So and I'll be looking after you today." (You'll hear that one, for sure.)

So, what's behind that "Dr." proclamation? Are all doctors made equal?

That's not really a fair question. A physician grows as a professional in the same way other professionals do—they begin with a foundation of knowledge (from their formal training) and grow in proficiency and wisdom as the years of experience add up. As with anyone else, some grow more than others.

Why do I bring this up? For you, dear reader, as you should know that differences exist in skill and competence of physicians and surgeons—and respiratory therapists, physiotherapists, dieticians, and so on… and experience weighs heavily on the development of these skills. There are a few simple categories to understand the stages through which doctors can progress—other paths exist, of course, but these are the main ones. Let's start at the beginning of when "Dr." enters the vocabulary.

Medical Students

These are students in medical school *training* to become a medical doctor. They are required to spend time in various parts of the hospital learning the basics of many different fields of medicine.

Following graduation from a medical school, they are now considered medical doctors. But they're not able to independently practice medicine yet… they are, however, eligible to begin a residency program and become medical residents (also known as *interns*).

Medical Residents

These are doctors who have finished medical school and are undergoing the their on-the-job apprenticeship for their chosen field (to become an anesthesiologist, for example). This can take two to six years to complete, depending on the field they pursue.

After completing residency and sitting the required regulatory exams, these docs are ready to go. Fly little bird, fly! Interestingly, I've had some anesthesiologists just starting their first job tell me that it's both exciting and a little scary to be fully on their own. Until now, they've had teachers and mentors guiding them for the better part of 10 years. They are well prepared but know they still have a lot to learn.

Clinical Fellows

These are experienced doctors who are pursuing further specialty training (called a *fellowship*) in their chosen field, such as paediatric cardiac surgery (heart surgery for kids). Some of these folks just can't get enough—you'll find some of them working on their Masters or PhD simultaneously... God love them.

Staff Physicians and Surgeons

After their formal training (medical school, residency, +/- a fellowship) and passing regulatory exams, these doctors are prepared to support the hospital as a member of the medical or surgical staff (called *consultants* in some countries).

They are now the teachers, mentors and leaders. The weight of responsibility and decision rests with them daily—some days that weight is heavier than others but it is theirs to bear. This responsibility is what gives such weight to their title.

As a patient having surgery, you'll mainly be working with surgeons and anesthesiologists. In the next chapter, we'll discuss their roles in the context of your surgery.

Registered Nurses

Registered Nurses (RNs) have important roles in most areas of healthcare. Within the hospital setting, these professionals work in many different capacities with varying types of responsibilities, including direct patient care, leadership, research, education and hospital administration.

When it comes to your surgery, you'll work directly with nurses before, during and after your procedure. The nursing profession proudly considers itself to be a strong patient advocate. I can say from experience that this advocacy is clearly an integral part of nursing practice—not only am I married to a nurse, I've worked with many nurses that I'd consider role models of how to put the patient first. This philosophy has directly influenced the creation of this book—remember, you are the most important part of your care (as you may recall from the Introduction).

Allied Health Professionals

Allied health professionals include a large variety of providers that have very specialized training and expertise. Together, allied health professionals, doctors and nurses combine to create dynamic and creative healthcare teams. We'll cover some of these professionals in more detail a little later. For now, here's a snapshot of these professionals:

ALLIED HEALTH PROFESSIONALS	
▶ ANESTHESIA ASSISTANTS	▶ OCCUPATIONAL THERAPISTS
▶ AUDIOLOGISTS	▶ PHARMACISTS
▶ BIOETHICISTS	▶ PHYSIOTHERAPISTS
▶ CARDIOVASCULAR PERFUSIONISTS	▶ PSYCHOLOGISTS
▶ CHIROPODISTS	▶ RADIATION THERAPISTS
▶ KINESIOLOGISTS	▶ REGISTERED DIETICIANS
▶ LABORATORY MEDICINE PROFESSIONALS	▶ RESPIRATORY THERAPISTS
▶ MEDICAL IMAGING TECHNOLOGISTS	▶ SOCIAL WORKERS
▶ NURSE PRACTITIONERS	▶ SPEECH LANGUAGE PATHOLOGISTS
▶ NURSES	▶ SPIRITUAL CARE PROFESSIONALS

Quite a few, isn't it? I happen to fall into the "Anesthesia Assistants" and "Respiratory Therapists" categories.

Not all professions will be represented in every hospital. Regardless of who you meet—doctor, nurse, social worker, etc.—these professionals are not only well trained, they also have standards to which they must adhere. Most health professions are regulated, meaning that the scope of their practice is well defined and they are accountable for their actions and interactions with patients and other professionals.

Healthcare professionals have earned and enjoy a lot of autonomy in their work. With this comes a responsibility to uphold a pre-defined standard of practice.

Support Staff

Some of the most caring, charismatic and supportive people I've met in healthcare were members of the support staff that work together with the professionals previously mentioned. They work to ensure your stay at the hospital is safe, comfortable, clean (really clean), timely and efficient.

Here are some examples of support staff you may meet in the hospital:

- Personal Support Workers
- Patient Care Aids
- Porters
- Operating Room Attendants

Hospital Administration & Office Staff

From the Chief Executive Officer (CEO), Chief Financial Officer (CFO), and Vice Presidents to clinic administrative staff, these people work to ensure your stay meets or exceeds established standards for patient care.

The administrative staff you are most likely to encounter are the people who greet you at the Pre-Admission Clinic, Laboratory Clinics (for any tests you might need) and the Pre-Operative Area. These staff will provide you with guidance and direction at each step along the way.

Hospital Board of Directors

While you are unlikely to meet a member of the Hospital Board during your stay, this group of highly skilled people from a variety of business and healthcare backgrounds have the job of holding the hospital to account by ensuring it is operating in a safe, effective, efficient and responsible manner. The hospital CEO reports to the Hospital Board (even the boss has a boss).

Volunteers

Sometimes walking into the lobby of a large hospital is overwhelming. Most hospitals have a large "Information" sign displayed near the main entrance. Here, a valuable group of people await to answer your questions and help you on your way. If you're not sure of your next step, this would be a good place to ask for help.

Volunteers often have important roles to play in hospital fundraising efforts as well. I've been a part of fundraising events in the past. It's a very rewarding way to get involved, give back to your hospital and meet some great people! Maybe volunteering at a hospital is in your future?

Oh, the Places You'll Go... The Flow of Your Hospital Stay

The type of surgery you are having will determine which areas of the hospital you will see. To get started, let's quickly walk through each area you'll typically encounter. In the next chapter, we'll discuss in more detail how you'll interact with each area on the day of surgery.

START HERE

Surgical Reception

This is typically where you will check in on the day of surgery. Be prepared to provide your identification, hospital card, insurance information and/or other paperwork.

Typically, you'll be shown to a change room to put on one of those elegant hospital gowns. It's a good idea to use the bathroom at this time too—you may not have another chance!

Pre-Operative Area

Next, you'll have a seat in the Pre-Operative Area. This is where you'll be interviewed by some of the healthcare professionals we talked about earlier. These people will be very interested in what you have to say! Expect to be asked questions more than once by different people—that's okay, this is truly for your safety. Everyone involved, including you, wants to make sure that the right person is getting the right surgery at the right time. Right?

Operating Room (OR)

My favourite place!

I spent many years working as a member of the Operating Room team. Sometimes, it's a fast-moving, dynamic and fun environment. At other times it has an incredible tension as exceptionally difficult and skillful work is being performed. Truly a rewarding environment in which to work.

As the person lying on the Operating Room table, you'll see things a little differently!

That's okay.

Just remember, you still have a voice here and should feel empowered to ask questions and participate in discussions. More on this in the next chapter.

Post-Anesthetic Care Unit (PACU)

Both the anesthetic and the surgery have elements that you will need to recover from. The Post-Anesthetic Care Unit is a space designed to allow you to recover while being closely monitored.

Pain control is an important element of the care in the PACU. This is a complicated and sophisticated field of medicine. More on pain control a little later too.

Intensive Care Unit (ICU)

This unit is reserved for critically ill patients and those requiring a high degree of monitoring and medical care following surgery. Patients in the ICU will generally receive one-to-one care by an ICU-trained Registered Nurse (RN).

Many patients in the ICU will also require mechanical ventilation (artificial support of their breathing) at some period during their admission. In North America, these patients are closely attended to by a Registered Respiratory Therapist (RRT).

Once a patient has been supported through their acute illness, injury or surgery, they will then be transferred to a Medical or Surgical Ward to continue their recovery.

Surgical Ward

If you'll be spending one or more nights recovering in hospital, you'll do so on the Surgical Ward. Important work is done here by a team of professionals to look after your pain control, mobility and readiness to go home.

💡 INSIDER TIP

The best time for you to ask any lingering questions is while you're in the Pre-Operative Area. Don't feel like you are being a bother. Your questions are important. Progressive hospitals will actively seek to involve you as a partner in all decisions surrounding your care. You have the right to be informed about your care and to ask for information and clarification about care being provided to you. Many hospitals have adopted a culture of Patient-Centred Care (PCC) that holds the patient as an active participant that is engaged in their healthcare.

At the same time, you also have a right to privacy. You will be asked to share very personal information and you should be able to do so in a way that maintains your confidentiality. Having privacy will allow you to share more easily. And share you should. Give complete answers to the questions you are asked, even if it may be uncomfortable. Incomplete information makes it difficult to optimize the care you are given.

Your family and friends can play a very valuable role here in helping you recover, stay comfortable and communicate and advocate for your needs. Get them involved!

Now that you've organized your trip to the hospital and have been introduced to those you'll be working with once you get there, let's dive into the day itself—the day of surgery.

3

THE DAY OF SURGERY

PURPOSE OF THIS CHAPTER
To give you clarity as to what happens on the day of surgery, ensure you're prepared and give you the confidence to participate actively.

KEY THINGS WE'LL COVER
- Your first steps of the day (including the night before)
- How your prep work will pay off
- You and the OR
- The people and things that keep you safe
- The experience of anesthesia—going to sleep and waking up
- What to expect immediately after surgery

LET'S BEGIN WITH the night before...

Nice work so far. You've done (hopefully) a lot of preparation. Let's review what you've taken care of already:

- You've educated yourself about your **health and medications**
- You've come to understand **your role as a patient** and have expectations to **participate actively** in your care
- You've **learned about your hospital** and how you'll move through it
- **You've gotten organized!** (*hospital & travel; surgery & appointments; health & medications; recovery & questions*)

Now, here we are on the night before your surgery. You might be nervous—perhaps feeling a little jittery. That's completely normal. Aside from these normal jitters though, your preparation has given you a much better understanding of what parts of this process you can control—and you've taken big steps to take control of these. All your efforts have set you up for a successful outcome. The day of surgery will be largely about allowing the skill of your healthcare providers to be put into action.

Everyone's goal is to achieve the best possible outcome for *you*. There will be times during the day of surgery where your job will be to trust in others and allow the professionals to do their work (you're not totally off the hook though—more on this later).

Remember that piece we touched on earlier about acceptance and gratitude? This mindset can be helpful the night before and the day of surgery. Don't wish the situation to be different than it is (it can't be, of course). Be mindful of your inner dialogue—the words you tell yourself profoundly influence how you experience a situation.

You'll have more work to do in the morning but not tonight. You're ready. Set your alarm and get a good night's sleep. See you in the morning…

> 📣 **CALL TO ACTION**
>
> Here are your tasks on the night before surgery:
>
> 1. Review your Ready for My Surgery Checklist (is everything you need to bring organized and packed up?)
> 2. Review instructions from your surgeon and anesthesiologist (when to stop eating and drinking, medications to take (or not), etc.)
> 3. Connect with the person accompanying you to the hospital
> 4. Unwind in whatever healthy way works for you
> 5. Sleep well (Tip: If your mind starts getting busy, focus your attention on your breathing—it's boring… eventually you'll fall asleep!)

The Morning of Surgery

Eating and Drinking Before Surgery

Let's start with this topic—it affects everyone going for surgery and it's commonly misunderstood. Everyone going for an elective surgery is told a time after which they should not eat or drink (i.e. the fasting period).

So, what's the big deal about eating and drinking before surgery?

Well… what goes down, *could* come back up.

Before I explain this further, if you are sensitive to "gross" topics, go ahead and skip the next paragraph and just take my word that following instructions related to eating and drinking before surgery is really important. If you'd like to know why, read on!

We've all lost our lunch during a bout of the flu. The good thing, I suppose, is that we're conscious during these unpleasant episodes of vomiting and can manage the process. Things change under anesthesia—you'll be unconscious or less conscious and consequently unable to "protect your airway," as anesthesia-types will say. What does that mean? It means that people under general anesthesia cannot prevent regurgitated stomach contents from entering their lungs (this is called aspiration*). Stomach contents are bad for the lungs—they are acidic, maybe chunky (nasty) and ultimately can cause widespread inflammation of the lung tissue (think of it like burning your skin with a chemical). Through this inflammation, aspiration of stomach contents can lead to further injury of the lungs (primarily, impairing their ability to allow oxygen to enter your blood) and can require a longer length of stay in hospital and more invasive interventions to help with recovery (such as being on a mechanical ventilator). This is the basis for the guidelines on eating and drinking before surgery.*

SHOW ME THE EVIDENCE

FASTING BEFORE SURGERY

Guidelines published on the duration of fasting before surgery by the American Society of Anesthesiologists and the Canadian Anesthesiologists' Society are based on a comprehensive review of the available research. Here's the duration of fasting recommended by anesthesiologists for healthy patients of any age having an elective surgery:[1]

- 8 hours: After eating meat, fried or fatty foods
- 6 hours: After a light meal (e.g. toast), infant formula or milk
- 4 hours: After breast milk
- 2 hours: After clear fluids (e.g. water, clear tea, black coffee (sugar is okay but 6 hours with cream), carbonated drinks and fruit juice without pulp—no alcohol though!)

Why be so specific? Why not just tell everyone to stop eating and drinking after midnight? A few reasons:

1. To prevent unnecessary dehydration
2. To prevent low blood sugar levels (called *hypoglycemia*)
3. To improve your comfort and experience with surgery

Certain conditions can change fasting recommendations. Some examples include diabetes, obesity, pregnancy, gastroesophageal reflux disease (GERD, or acid reflux) and emergency surgery.

Ask your surgeon and anesthesiologist what specific guidelines apply to you. Eat well and stay hydrated in the days leading up to your surgery. Keep it up until the deadline given to you—they should be close to what we've covered here unless you have a condition that increases your risk of an associated complication.

---

1 "Practice Guidelines for Preoperative Fasting and the Use of Pharmacologic Agents to Reduce the Risk of Pulmonary Aspiration." *Anesthesiology* (2017), https://anesthesiology.pubs.asahq.org/article.aspx?articleid=2596245.

Morning Check—Your Ready for My Surgery Checklist

On the morning of surgery, peek at your Ready for My Surgery Checklist and be sure to bring it with you. The main things you need to bring are listed here. You will have added to it as well during your preparation. Here are the key sections of the checklist to review before leaving for the hospital:

- *Day of Surgery*
- *Other Things to Bring*

Note: Pay special attention to the instructions given to you by your surgeon

Ready? Time to hit the road.

You've Arrived

Okay, good, you've made it to the hospital on time. Early, you say? Even better. You've got all your stuff and know where you're going too, that's good (if you need a reminder of where to go, remember the folks at the Information desk).

Now, you'll make your way to Surgical Reception where you will check in for your procedure. Thank goodness you had prepared all your paperwork in advance, it's the first thing they ask for!

The clerk at the Surgical Reception desk will ensure you are in the right place, have all required documentation and will help you with your initial preparation. This may include changing your clothes into a hospital gown and managing your personal belongings.

Pre-Operative Area

From the reception area, you'll then make your way to a Pre-Operative (meaning, "before surgery") Area where additional preparation is done prior to heading into the Operating Room. This space has different names in different hospitals but the key is that there is generally a place where you will wait before going into the OR. The following narrative will give you a sense of what happens here.

Picture This
Imagine yourself hopping up on a small bed, called a stretcher (though sometimes it's just a chair). You then take notice of a couple (yup, Steve and Mary) in the bed

space next to you. They arrived just a few moments earlier. You can overhear their conversation...

"THESE GOWNS ARE flattering," Mary says sarcastically.

"Busy place in here," says Steve as he looks around the room, seemingly unaware of Mary's comment. He's a little surprised at how full of people and activity it is for 7:00 a.m.

Mary and Steve watch the people in hospital scrubs walk hurriedly past their little bed space. Some have those lightweight OR hats on, some don't. One fellow walks by with a hat on but is clearly bald—Steve doesn't understand this entirely.

"You should go for a walk or something while I'm in there. The operation is supposed to take a few hours," Mary says as she fidgets with the new ID band around her wrist. She looks up and sees a woman in scrubs heading her way.

"Hi there, how are you today?" the woman says as she smiles and acknowledges both Mary and Steve.

"Fine, thank you," Mary replies.

"My name is Nicole. I'm a nurse and I'll be checking you in." Nicole picks up the beginnings of a chart off the table at the foot of Mary's bed and begins scanning through it.

"May I see your wristband?" she asks.

"Of course," Mary says.

"Thanks. What is your full name?" the nurse asks as she reads the name printed on Mary's ID band.

"Mary King—and this is my husband, Steve. Not the author of course, in case you were wondering—*his* books scare me," she says.

"I'm sure he'd be happy to hear that," Nicole laughs. "Would you tell me your date of birth?"

"September 19th, 1953," Mary offers.

"Great. And what surgery are you having today?"

"It's called a coronary bypass, I believe—heart surgery," Mary says.

"Is this your signature on the consent form?" Nicole asks as she shows Mary the piece of paper.

"It is."

"Thank you very much. What did you have for breakfast today, Mary?" Nicole asks.

"Oh, I wasn't supposed to eat this morning. The last thing I had was a glass of water before bed at about 10 o'clock."

"Excellent, thank you," Nicole says with a smile. "Do you have any allergies?"

"No," says Mary.

"Has anyone come by to put a mark on your skin where the surgery will be?"

"Yes, a young doctor was here just before you and she signed her initials on my chest," Mary says as she shows Nicole the mark.

"Okay, then. Do you have any questions or concerns about your procedure today?" asks Nicole.

"Not yet," Mary says.

"Well, be sure to let me know if you do. Now, I'd like to quickly take your temperature, blood pressure and check the oxygen level in your blood with a little sensor, is that okay?" Nicole says as she wheels the vital signs monitor over to the side of Mary's bed.

"Sure, no problem," says Mary.

Steve watches with interest as the blood pressure cuff is wrapped around Mary's upper arm. The nurse pushes a button and the cuff starts to inflate like a balloon. He can tell that it's pretty tight by the look on Mary's face but it quickly deflates and leaves a blood pressure measurement on the monitor screen.

"Is that blood pressure okay?" asks Steve.

"It's a little high," says Nicole. "But it's pretty common for your blood pressure to be higher than usual right before surgery—a lot of people are a little nervous."

"Mine's probably high too," Steve laughs as he looks at Mary. "The drive in here didn't help."

SO, WHAT HAPPENED *here?*

A few important things, it turns out:

- Nicole identified herself as a nurse
- The patient's identification was verified
- The type of surgery described by Mary was consistent with the OR booking
    - *Is there a guarantee that the OR booking is correct? No, there isn't ... Take the time to clarify that your understanding of the procedure exactly matches theirs*
- Nicole verified that Mary had signed consent for the procedure
- Nicole made sure that Mary had nothing to eat or drink that morning

- Nicole asked Mary if there was anything she'd like to discuss (an act of including the patient in their care—something you should expect)

- Baseline vital sign measurements were taken. Mary's temperature, blood pressure, heart rate and oxygen saturation would be recorded in her chart (i.e. medical record). Nicole would have also silently counted Mary's respiratory (breathing) rate while the blood pressure measurement was being taken.

Can you expect something similar? Most definitely. These are the key things that need to be verified at the start. If anything differs from expectations (yours or theirs), the time to sort it out is now.

Is a mistake possible at this stage? Mistakes are possible at any stage. However, each exchange you have with professionals on the day of surgery is an opportunity to make sure everyone is on the same page.

Similar to Mary, you'll be asked a number of questions by an RN when you arrive to the Pre-Operative Area. Remember, you should *expect* to be asked the same questions multiple times by different people—this is just the first round.

Ask Your Own Questions

As we've already covered, it's ideal to have most of your questions and concerns addressed before the day of surgery. However, if you have a question or concern about anything—even if you think it is NOT important—it is important! Don't hesitate to ask to speak with your surgeon. They need *you* to be clear on what is about to happen and why.

By now, I'm sure you appreciate just how valuable your preparation could become. The questions so far have been easy…

Other Things to Come in the Pre-Operative Area

There is more that could be covered with you than was asked of Mary during this example conversation. Much of this depends on the surgery you're having and your state of health. For more complex surgeries, such as Mary's heart surgery, it's very likely that you'll have blood samples taken ahead of time for analysis. If your surgical team has been monitoring any particular blood values, they may need to check on these again on the morning of surgery.

🔍 SHOW ME THE EVIDENCE

BLOOD TRANSFUSIONS

Blood transfusions during surgery can be life-saving and when needed, the benefits most likely outweigh the risks.

BENEFITS OF A TRANSFUSION

Doctors will only give you a blood transfusion if absolutely necessary. If you've lost blood during surgery and you're in a situation where the volume of your blood (or a component of it) is low, a transfusion can help with:

- Increasing the number of red blood cells (these carry oxygen to your body's cells—essential for life)

- Increasing blood clotting components (especially vital for someone having surgery)

- Increasing circulating blood volume (an average adult has about 5 litres of blood being pumped through their body by their heart—without enough volume, the heart can't pump properly)

RISKS OF A TRANSFUSION

Having a reaction from a blood transfusion is unlikely but there are some known risks. These risks should be explained to you ahead of time so that you can make an informed decision. To prepare you for that conversation, here are some risks you should be aware of:

MOST COMMON REACTIONS:
- Allergic reaction (e.g. itching; hives—an antihistamine usually looks after this)

- Fever and chills (typically within four hours of the transfusion)

RARE REACTIONS:
- Blood infection (e.g. in 2015, reported rates were 1 in 21.4 million for an HIV infection and 1 in 12.6 for Hepatitis C in Canada)[2]

- Destruction of the new red blood cells by the recipient's body

- Injury to the lungs or difficulty breathing

- A condition where the new white blood cells attack bone marrow

Due to the known risks and the high value of donated blood, transfusions are only performed if necessary. Your surgeon and anesthesiologist will help you understand how this topic applies to your situation.

---

2 Canadian Blood Services Surveillance Report, 2015, https://blood.ca/sites/default/files/External_Surveillance_Report_2015.pdf.

Here are a few other activities that could take place before going into the OR:

- An intravenous (IV) catheter may be placed. IVs are usually inserted into a vein in the back of your hand or your arm—this is where most of the medications and fluids will be administered.

- Blood tests are sometimes required, such as for blood glucose levels for people with diabetes.

- Some people will need breathing tests performed (called *bedside spirometry*).

The theme of all the activities in the Pre-Operative Area is *readiness*. Your anesthesia, surgical and nursing teams will all be making sure you're ready. Each will have their particular focus as they speak with you. Let's tackle the surgeons first.

Surgeons in the Pre-Operative Area

Before having you transferred into the OR, here are your surgeon's main goals:

- Verify with you the type and location of your surgery
- Ensure you have signed the consent form for the procedure (meaning that you thoroughly understand what you've signed up for—this is called *informed consent*)
- Ensure you have followed your pre-surgery instructions
- Mark the site of surgery on your skin
- When required, discuss the possibility of a blood transfusion during surgery (if there is a risk of blood loss during surgery that would require a blood transfusion)

> ## 💡 INSIDER TIP
>
> **PRE-OPERATIVE AREA: THE WAITING PLACE**
>
> Let's face it, waiting in the Pre-Operative Area is just the appetizer—the prelude—to the feature event. It is, however, a place where you may first start feeling uneasy (if you hadn't already!). Now, it's on. You're in a hospital gown with nothing but your birthday suit underneath and the flurry of activity has begun.
>
> **TAKE A DEEP BREATH**
>
> Know that you're ready. You have prepared well—you've done your part up to now. In this short period before you go into the Operating Room, your job is simply to stay alert to the numerous questions and instructions you are given. It's a conversation—engage in it.

Correct Patient, Correct Site, Correct Procedure

Are you crystal clear on the surgical procedure you are having and exactly where on your body the operation will take place? You need to be. This is one of the most important tasks you have on the day of surgery.

Be clear with every person you speak to on:
1. *The type of surgery you are having*
2. *The site(s) on your body on which it is to take place*

There are a number of places where miscommunication can occur regarding your procedure, especially if it is a procedure that could be performed on the right or left side of the body (e.g. knee, hand, kidney, etc.).

If the World Health Organization (WHO) thinks it a big deal, we should too. Below are some snippets from the WHO Guidelines for Safe Surgery. I've selected pieces that really stand out from a patient perspective. If you'd like to read more, you can find the entire document at www.who.int/patientsafety/safesurgery/.

> **SHOW ME THE EVIDENCE**
>
> **CORRECT SITE SURGERY**
> The World Health Organization created a document called WHO Guidelines for Safe Surgery: Safe Surgery Saves Lives. There is one section in particular that is worth us spending a little time on, it's entitled "The team will operate on the correct patient at the correct site."
>
> Here, the WHO highlights an estimated 1,500–2,500 incidents of surgery being performed on either the wrong patient or on the wrong part of the patient's body in the United States each year. That's a rate of one such error in 50,000–100,000 surgeries. The risk is higher for surgeries that can be done on either the right or left side (i.e. you have two hips but only one heart).
>
> Maybe you didn't really want to know that. But here's why I think you do:
>
> Among the key recommendations to reduce this risk are patient involvement in planning for your surgery, as well as informed consent.
>
> Your participation matters.
>
> A lot of work has been done to reduce the risk of errors during surgery, yet work remains. The more you think of yourself as a vital, active member of your health-care team, the greater the potential for you to positively influence the safety of your care.

Your Safety Is Your Job Too

Before reading this book, you may not have appreciated this statement—I'm sure you do now. Think of this next section as a job description. You have a role as part of this team. Here's how it should work.

The World Health Organization's Universal Protocol

This protocol was designed to make sure the correct patient gets the correct surgical procedure on the correct site of their body. I've listed the three steps for you—but more importantly, highlighted how you can actively participate in each one:

1. Verification

YOUR TEAM'S JOB: Clinicians will verify with one another the correct patient, site and procedure any time your care is transferred from one person to another.

YOUR JOB: You should verify with your healthcare team the type and location of your surgery at the time your surgery is scheduled, when you're admitted to hospital, during your Pre-Operative Area check-in, when you sign consent for the procedure and in the Operating Room.

2. Marking

YOUR TEAM'S JOB: Someone from the surgical team (resident, fellow, staff surgeon) will spend some time with you. Even though you will likely be nervous, it is very important that you give those moments your full attention. They will place a mark on your skin where the surgery is to be performed, typically with a pen or marker. To ensure the mark is made in the correct place, they will verify with you the type and location of surgery—be engaged in this part of the process. This is one of the important things that the RN working with you in the Pre-Operative Area will be looking for. In most hospitals, if there's no mark the surgical team will be called to do this before you are taken into the OR.

YOUR JOB: Make sure the correct site is being marked! The WHO says, *"... marking must be ... completed, to the extent possible, while the patient is alert and awake, as the patient's involvement is important."*[3]

3. Time Out

YOUR TEAM'S JOB: You'll actually be asleep during the "Time Out" or "Surgical Pause" that takes place just before the surgery begins. However, before you are given an anesthetic, there is a briefing called the "Sign In" during which you *should* be asked to participate.

YOUR JOB: Participate during the "Sign In" discussion about your surgery that occurs once you are in the OR (more on this later).

To be clear, the reason this protocol was developed is because errors do happen. **"The Joint Commission views failure to engage the patient (or his or her caregiver) as one of the causes of wrong-site surgery."**[4]

As a patient already engaged in this process, *you* have the power to make up for such failures! Demand to be engaged—it's your right. As it turns out, there is evidence that **your participation can prevent an error in your surgery.**

MOVING ON.

So far, we've met the Pre-Operative Area RN and sorted out the details of your surgery with the surgical team. Now it's time to meet the Anesthesia Team.

---

3   WHO Guidelines for Safe Surgery: Safe Surgery Saves Lives, 2009, World Health Organization, https://www.who.int/patientsafety/safesurgery/tools_resources/9789241598552/en/.

4   WHO Guidelines for Safe Surgery: Safe Surgery Saves Lives, 2009, World Health Organization, https://www.who.int/patientsafety/safesurgery/tools_resources/9789241598552/en/.

Anesthesia Care Team

Let's start with a couple of common questions:

    Who are anesthetists? What *exactly* do they do?

    But wait, aren't they called anesthesiologists? They're doctors, right?

If you're not clear on this, you're not alone. Here's a piece from the newsletter of the Canadian Anesthesiologists' Society. They see this as a problem (and it is) so let's take this opportunity to get the two of you acquainted.

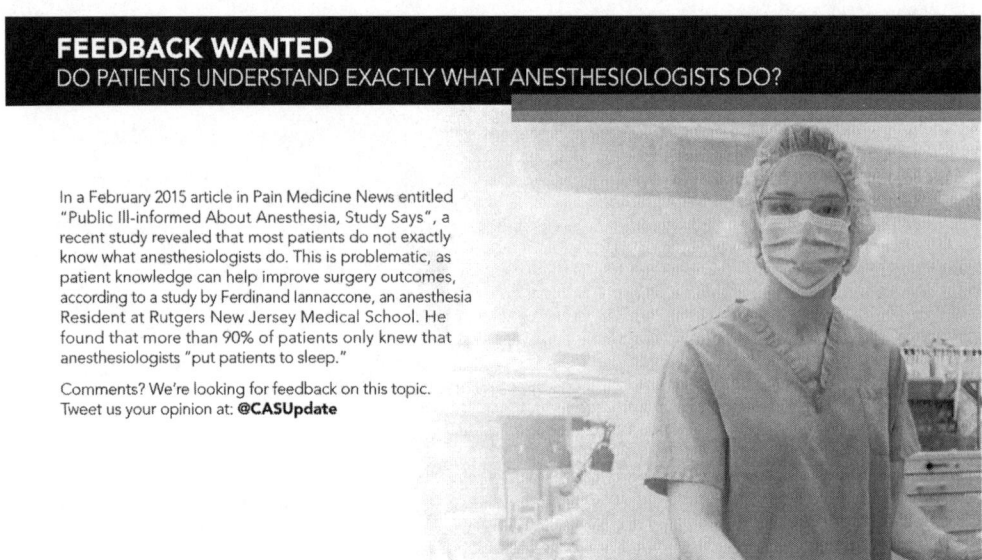

Canadian Anesthesiologists' Society Newsletter, Volume 30, Number 2—June 2015. Feedback Wanted: Do Patients Understand Exactly What Anesthesiologists Do? Retrieved February 24, 2017 with permission.

    Trust me, you want to know what they do—and it's probably more than you think. If you don't meet someone from the Anesthesia Team at a Pre-Admission Clinic visit, you'll certainly meet one of the team at some point ahead of your surgery. So, let's briefly unpack the titles of anesthesiologist, anesthetist, nurse anesthetist and anesthesia assistant.

Meet the Anesthesia Team

*Anesthesiologist [an-es-thee-zee-**ol**-***uh***-*jist*]*

Sure, it's a bit of a tongue twister but this doctor has earned a lot of letters after their name. With around 10 years of medical training, physician anesthesiologists have an enormous breadth and depth of medical knowledge. I've worked closely with these professionals for many years and I have the utmost respect for the profession and the skillful and vigilant care they provide.

In a nutshell, anesthesiologists provide complete care of patients immediately before, during and after surgery. This includes:

- Assessing your state of health prior to surgery, including any medical conditions
- Creating and implementing a plan for your anesthetic based on this assessment, the type of surgery you're having and their discussion with you about your preferences
- Monitoring and managing your vital signs throughout the surgery
- Supporting your recovery from the anesthetic, including pain control

Complex anesthetic care. The extensive training of anesthesiologists prepares them to manage the most challenging patient and surgical scenarios. Many further their training to sub-specialize in areas such as cardiac anesthesia, thoracic (lung) anesthesia and neuroanesthesia (anesthesia care for surgeries on the brain and spinal cord).

Leaders. Anesthesiologists are the leaders of Anesthesia Care Teams in environments where there is a multi-disciplinary approach to anesthesia care. Even when an anesthetic is being provided by a non-physician clinician, anesthesiologists provide close consultation and are at the ready to provide direct assistance when needed.

GP-Anesthetist [a-nes-thi-tist]

Some family doctors (General Practitioners) undergo specialty training in anesthesia to become GP-Anesthetists. Many Community Hospitals employ GP-Anesthetists to provide anesthesia care for their surgical patients. Typically, the practice of GP-Anesthetists will be limited to common surgeries on relatively healthy patients where a complex anesthetic and monitoring regimen is not required.

Anesthesia Assistant (AA)

A profession near and dear to my heart! After training and practicing as a Respiratory Therapist, I pursued specialty training as an Anesthesia Assistant and enjoyed many years of challenging and rewarding work as part of an Anesthesia Care Team.

AAs are non-physician anesthesia care providers that *work with* anesthesiologists in many different practice settings. Anesthesia Assistants are skilled healthcare professionals that come from a variety of professional backgrounds—typically nursing and respiratory therapy in Canada, for example. Should you be fortunate enough to have an AA look after you for your anesthetic, you would be in great hands.

Certified Registered Nurse Anesthetist (CRNA)

CRNAs are anesthesia specialists with a scope of practice similar to the Anesthesia Assistant. These non-physician anesthesia care providers practice anesthesia in the United States and many other countries, but not in Canada. They're highly trained through a graduate nursing program and have been around a long time—about 150 years.

Pre-Operative Anesthesia Team Activities

Given all that was just covered on anesthesia professionals, you'll not be surprised that they too will have a number of questions when they meet you in the Pre-Operative Area. Even if you had met someone from the Anesthesia Team during a Pre-Admission Clinic visit, you may very well have someone different looking after you on the day of surgery.

As luck would have it, I've been in the position of the one asking the questions. So, it was easy for me to organize most of what you'll need to know into your Ready for My Surgery Checklist. The "My Health" section of the checklist contains most of the information anesthesia care providers will be seeking from you.

Quite often, a detailed review of your health is performed during the Pre-Admission Clinic visit we talked about in Chapter 1. If you didn't have this assessment, it will need to be done in the Pre-Operative Area. Either way, I encourage you to complete the "Medical Conditions" section of your checklist beforehand to help you give clearer and more complete answers. To make it easier, use the following as a reference for the types of conditions that are important for your care team to know about:

BODY SYSTEM	COMMON CONDITIONS
YOUR HEART (cardiovascular)	• High blood pressure • High cholesterol • Previous heart attacks, chest pain, heart surgery • Irregular heartbeats, pacemaker/defibrillator
YOUR LUNGS (respiratory)	• Smoking history • Asthma • Chronic obstructive pulmonary disease (COPD)—includes chronic bronchitis and emphysema • Other lung disease • Sleep apnea
YOUR GUT (gastrointestinal, renal, hepatic)	• Acid reflux (GERD) • Ulcer or bleeding from your stomach • Difficulty swallowing • Kidney disorders • Liver disease (e.g. hepatitis, jaundice, cirrhosis)
YOUR HORMONES (endocrine)	• Diabetes (type and control) • Thyroid disorder • Obesity • Medical steroid/cortisone use
YOUR NERVOUS SYSTEM (neurological)	• Stroke or "mini stroke" (called a *transient ischemic attack*—TIA) • Seizures • Neuropathy (e.g. numbness, weakness or paralysis) • Back or neck pain • Neuromuscular disease • Depression or anxiety • Memory problems (e.g. Alzheimer's, dementia) • Parkinson's disease
YOUR BLOOD (hematological)	• Bleeding problems (e.g. clotting disorders) • History of blood clots (e.g. pulmonary embolism, deep vein thrombosis (DVT)) • Sickle cell trait or disease • Previous blood transfusion
OTHER SYSTEMS (othertological ☺)	• Arthritis • Cancer • Pregnancy • Alcohol or recreational substance use • Chronic pain • Poor vision/hearing • Infectious disease • Dental work/issues

> **💡 INSIDER TIP**
>
> **BOOKING YOUR SURGERY**
>
> If it were me having surgery, I'd ask my surgeon (or the secretary that books his/her surgeries) to avoid being the last case of the day. This is the one that is most likely to be cancelled due to ORs running late.

The anesthesia care provider will ask to have a look inside your mouth. What they can or can't see tells them a lot about how easy it will be to manage your airway after they administer the anesthetic. In addition to checking out your oral structures (including your teeth), they'll assess how wide you can open your mouth and determine if you have any issues with your neck. This is all in an effort to assess if they should anticipate any difficulties placing a breathing tube should they need to do so.

There are a number of challenging questions you'll need to answer—good thing you'll be ready for them! Be sure to mention if there have been any significant changes to your health since your Pre-Operative Clinic visit, including new diagnoses, new medications or medication changes, new allergies, or new infections (such a cold or fever). Remember, if there is anything during these conversations that you don't understand, ask for clarification (if I seem to be repeating myself, it's on purpose). In order to make informed decisions, you need to understand what will happen and why, as well as the risks involved—this is the nature of informed consent.

Delays

Before we talk about the OR itself, let's briefly cover some of the barriers to you getting in there on time.

Operating Room time is expensive—some costing $100 per minute or more... Per *minute*.[5]

This creates a large incentive for Operating Room managers to balance the maximization of OR usage with keeping rooms running on schedule and finishing on time. Despite the best efforts of the whole team, unexpected delays can happen for a variety of reasons—surgical challenges, equipment issues, slow room turnover (the cleaning and preparation of the OR between surgeries) and emergencies.

As far as the clinicians are concerned, it's not costs that they're thinking about, it's efficiency. It's also that last patient of the day. Working hard to keep the OR running smoothly and on time will make sure that the room doesn't run over its allowable time limit. A late room means overtime pay for staff. Paying people overtime on a regular basis means that the budget for the OR also goes over. Be it a privately- or publicly-funded hospital, regular inefficiency leads to financial challenges and there are people held accountable for this. As such, many ORs are not

---

5 Alex Macario, "What Does One Minute of Operating Room Time Cost?" *Journal of Clinical Anesthesia* (2010), https://doi.org/10.1016/j.jclinane.2010.02.003.

permitted to run overtime. If insufficient time remains for the last case to finish on time, the last case may be cancelled.

Now a special note here: The OR in a hospital never fully closes, allowing for emergency surgeries at any time. I will assume that you are not reading this just prior to an emergency surgery!

Ready to Go

You're now told that it's time to make your way into the Operating Room (hopefully, no delays!). By this time:

- The Operating Room has been set up for your procedure
- The team has completed their pre-operative routine with you
- You have had a chance to ask any questions you may have

By foot, wheelchair or stretcher you'll travel to the Operating Room. You'll be joined by a member of the OR team—an OR nurse, the surgeon, a member of the Anesthesia Team and sometimes an OR attendant as well. Talking with the person that is accompanying you is a great way to keep from getting too nervous.

The Operating Room

The Centre of Attention

That's you! You are the most important person in the OR—yes, even more than the surgeon—and you should be treated that way.

Overwhelmed? Maybe Not Anymore

This is a common and understandable state for many people as they first walk into the Operating Room and lay down on the OR table (the fact that it's narrow and hard doesn't help). Your ability to accept the situation as it is really is one of the best ways to let go of your anxiety. Take a few slow, deep breaths if you need to—remember, it's okay and quite normal to feel nervous at this part of the process!

Trust is key and your healthcare team will hopefully have built some trust with you by this time. You can also trust that you've prepared well and this has set you up

> **INSIDER TIP**

EMERGENCY SURGERIES
Many University Teaching Hospitals are regional centres for certain types of specialty emergency surgeries, such as trauma and transplant surgery. Understanding the type of hospital that you are going to for surgery can help you understand the possibility of an emergency impacting you.

When someone requires emergency surgery, it is possible that a particular Operating Room and/or a particular surgeon, already performing elective surgeries, will need to be utilized for the emergency. This can lead to the cancellation of some cases—it could include yours.

Healthcare providers understand that this can be quite frustrating and inconvenient and so they are usually good at delivering such news with compassion.

A good way to look at it: Consider yourself or a loved one as being the person in need of emergency surgery and being grateful to the people who made room so you could receive the care you urgently required.

for a successful outcome. You have the knowledge, understanding and confidence to lay back and allow the care you need to be performed. It should be comforting to know that your healthcare team is made up of people who have dedicated their professional lives to honing the skills required to provide this care. I'm proud to have been one of them.

Behind the Masks

Most of the OR professionals you'll meet have been through this hundreds, maybe thousands of times. You've been introduced to most of the professionals already, but let's recap the core team you'll likely meet when you enter the OR:

Anesthesia Team
- You'll have one or more of the anesthesia professionals we discussed earlier work with you in the OR. We'll go over more of their role a little later.

OR Nurses
SCRUB NURSE
- This person will set up the surgical instruments and then work together with the surgeon to provide an efficient flow of instruments as they are needed during surgery
- The Scrub Nurse will be in a sterile gown with gloves and a mask when you enter the room

CIRCULATING NURSE
- This nurse coordinates the flow and turnover of the OR, makes sure the team has everything they need and communicates to those outside the OR
- It's the Circulating Nurse that will most likely meet with you in the Pre-Operative Area and possibly accompany you into the OR

Surgical Team
SURGEON
- You may think that it would be obvious to expect to see your surgeon in the OR when you arrive, but this isn't always the case.
- If the Nursing or Anesthesia Team have preparatory work to do ahead of the surgical checklist and induction of anesthesia (i.e. the process of putting you to

sleep, or more accurately, rendering you unconscious), the surgeon may give them the time and space to do this and head into the OR only when their contribution to the process is required.

- Surgeons are busy people who often use their time between surgeries productively, such as dictating notes and/or following up with previous patients.

- You may also discover that one of your surgeon's trainees (described in the next section) is standing in for him/her. If this is the case, ask to see your surgeon if you are uncomfortable with only seeing the trainee or with anything being discussed without your surgeon present.

SURGICAL/FIRST ASSIST
- This individual is a skilled assistant to the surgeon. This person is generally another doctor or a nurse with advanced training for this role.

CARDIOVASCULAR PERFUSIONIST
- Certain surgeries, such as open heart surgery, may require your heart to be stopped (yes, stopped…) for a period of time so that the cardiac surgeon and his/her surgical team can repair or replace whatever part of your heart is causing you trouble.

- So, how does blood continue to flow in your body while your heart is stopped? That's where the Cardiovascular Perfusionist comes in. These healthcare professionals specialize in the complex task of managing blood flow, blood pressure, gas exchange, some anesthesia delivery and more to keep you alive while your heart is stopped. As you can imagine, this is a very technical and demanding job!

Students

There is the potential for you to work with students anywhere in the hospital—the OR is no exception. The most common students you'll see in the OR are:

- Medical Students
- Medical & Surgical Residents/Fellows
- Nursing & Allied Health Students (e.g. Respiratory Therapists or Perfusionists)

> **💡 INSIDER TIP**
>
> **A NOTE ON STUDENTS**
> Be curious, ask students about their chosen profession. It can be intimidating when students first begin to practice their new-found skills on real people! As a patient, it's important to know that students are always closely monitored by supervising professional staff to ensure their care is appropriate, accurate and professional.
>
> To be clear, it is your choice to allow a student to participate in your care. If you are comfortable supporting their training by consenting to receive their care, you have provided a great service to the future of an important part of the healthcare system.

Wired for Sound

Things start moving quickly now. The team knows that getting the surgery started on time is key to it finishing on time. So, they move fast to prepare you for the induction of anesthesia (putting you to sleep).

Monitoring your vital signs during surgery is one of the most important ways to determine how your body is handling the procedure and the anesthetic. The thing is, the plethora of monitors can make you feel a little like a science experiment! Let's see how things go for Mary as she enters the OR...

"COME ON IN, Mary," Julie says as she opens the Operating Room door. The nurse guides Mary to the OR table, keeping herself between the trays of surgical instruments and her patient.

Mary glances around the room. She can see only the smiling eyes of the person masked and gowned standing beside the instruments. "Hi, Mary," he says, "I'm John—I'm another nurse that will be assisting Dr. Meyer with your surgery."

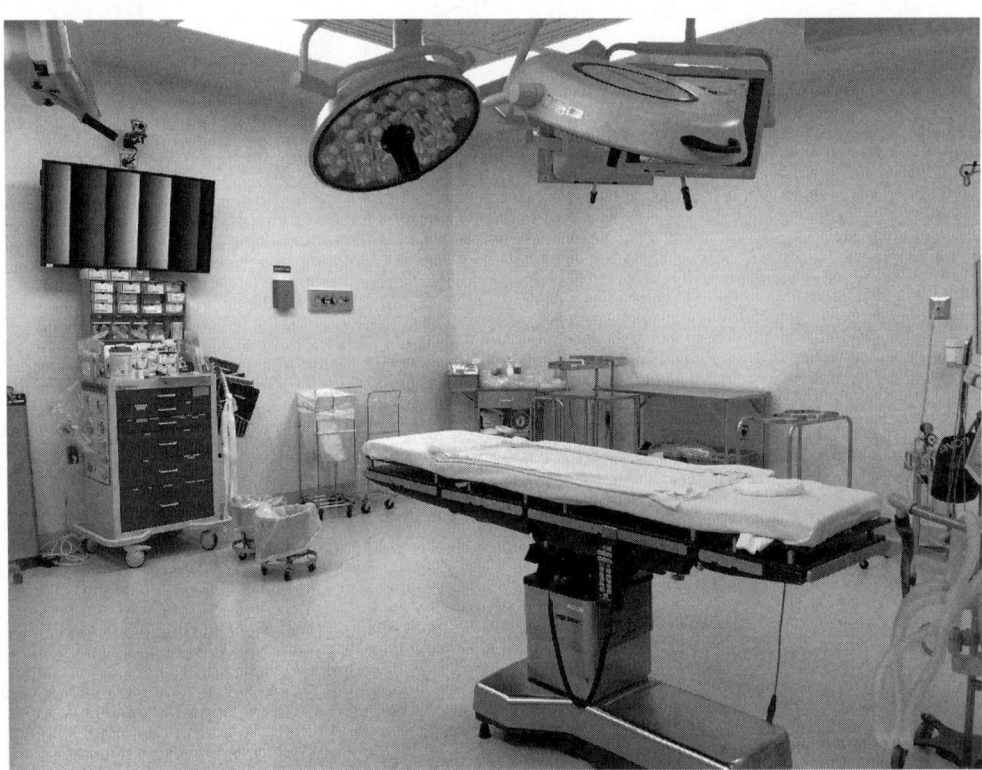

"Hi, John."

"Hop up on the table please, Mary—just be careful, it's a little narrow," Julie says.

Mary gets onto the OR table and is helped onto her back by Julie and Dr. Ryan, the anesthesiologist she'd met a little earlier the Pre-Operative Area. As she lays flat on the bed, he doubles up her pillow in an effort to make her a little more comfortable.

"Is that better?"

"Yes, much," says Mary. Though her neck is in a more comfortable position, she finds herself feeling quite vulnerable. She's very aware that she is wearing nothing beneath her light cotton gown. Mary also finds that having her arms outstretched by her sides on the arm boards attached to the OR table is uncomfortable and adds to her sense of vulnerability.

Large circular lights loom over Mary as she lays on the table. She recognizes these from the photos included in the material she read preparing for her surgery.

"Are you okay?" asks Julie.

"A little nervous," Mary confesses.

"That's very normal—don't worry, we're here to look after you," says Dr. Ryan, "We just have a few monitors to put on you, as well as an IV to start before putting you to sleep."

"This little clip goes on your finger," says Sam, "it measures the amount of oxygen in your blood."

A handful of round stickers are then placed on Mary's upper body and attached to small wires. *This is the ECG*, Mary thinks to herself—another tidbit gleaned from her reading.

"And this is a blood pressure cuff," says Dr. Ryan, "it's going to get pretty tight right now—it's always tightest when it takes the first blood pressure." Mary remembers this from the Pre-Operative Area; it seems a little tighter now though.

Before the blood pressure cuff finishes squeezing her right arm, Dr. Ryan approaches her left one with a long, blue rubber band in his hand.

"In the Pre-Operative Area, I mentioned that we'll need to start an IV. Would you mind if I do that now?" he asks.

"Of course," Mary says, "Will it hurt?"

"It's kind of like a bee sting," Dr. Ryan replies, "but I'll use some freezing medication so it's less painful."

"Thank you."

"You're welcome. Now, let's have a look—I'm just going to tap on the back of your hand to help the veins stand up better," Dr. Ryan says as he scours Mary's hand for a vein. "How are you doing?" he asks as he cleans a spot on the back of Mary's hand with an alcohol swab.

"Oh, peachy," says Mary sarcastically.

"This is going to sting a little," Dr. Ryan says as he quickly inserts the IV.

"There, it's done." He says, "the rest is much easier."

The OR door opens to Mary's right and Dr. Meyer, Mary's surgeon, walks in. He heads straight toward Mary.

"Hi, Mary, it's Dr. Meyer," he says, "are you all set?"

"As ready as I'll ever be."

"All right." Dr. Meyer asks the room, "Shall we do our Sign In?"

HOPEFULLY THIS COMMENTARY gives you a better idea of what you are likely to experience when you first enter the Operating Room. To give you a visual, here are a couple of photos of a typical OR.

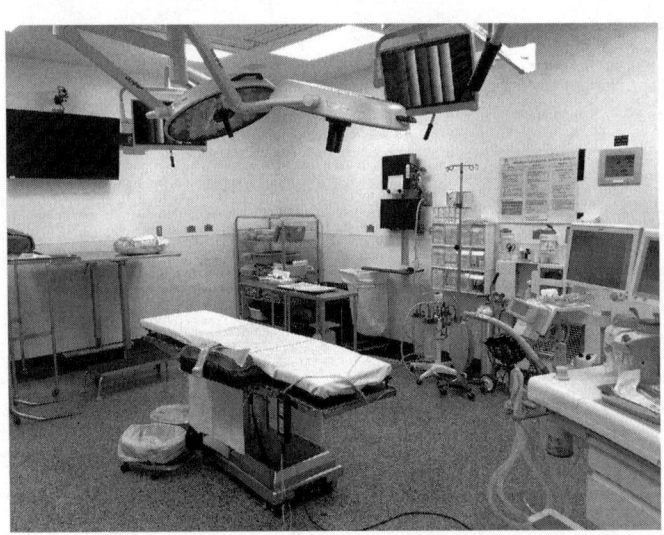
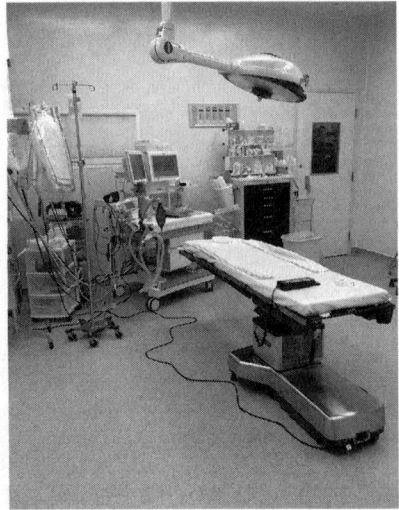

How You Are Monitored During Anesthesia

There are a few basic monitors used for every patient who receives an anesthetic. The essential ones are:

- Electrocardiogram (ECG/EKG)
- Pulse oximeter (a little clip placed over the tip of a finger that monitors the oxygen level in your blood).
- Blood pressure monitor

The description of these and other monitors can get a little technical and may not be of interest to everyone. For those who are interested in learning more, I've summarized each monitor in Appendix C. Please jump to that section at any time to explore these and other ways that clinicians keep an eye on you in the OR.

Your Safety

The World Health Organization's Surgical Safety Checklist
Remember the WHO's guidance around "correct site surgery" (correct patient, correct procedure, correct site)? Well, they're also front and centre when it comes to optimizing communication between members of the OR team on the most vital pieces of information pertaining to your surgery. Guess what they made… a checklist!

WHO doesn't like a checklist? ☺

Here's an excerpt:

The Checklist divides the operation into three phases, each corresponding to a specific time period in the normal flow of a procedure:

- *The period before induction of anesthesia ("Sign In")*
- *The period after induction and before surgical incision ("Time Out")*
- *The period during or immediately after wound closure but before removing the patient from the operating room ("Sign Out")*

In each phase, the Checklist coordinator must be permitted to confirm that the team has completed its tasks before it proceeds further.[6]

This was part of a groundbreaking initiative to improve the safety of surgical care worldwide. If you would like to learn more about this important work, visit the WHO website using the link in the footnote below.

How Will These Checklists Affect Me? (I Hear You Asking Yourself)
These checklists were designed to keep you safe during surgery.

You will be included in the first part of the checklist before you receive an anesthetic—speak up and make sure what is said matches your expectations! Ask for clarification if you need it, this is your right as a patient.

---

6 WHO Surgical Safety Checklist and Implementation Manual, 2008, World Health Organization, https://www.who.int/patientsafety/safesurgery/ss_checklist/en/.

Here's the first part of the checklist modified for you—it's called the "Sign In":

SIG N IN—BEFORE THE ANESTHETIC IS GIVEN[7]

☐ The patient (that's you) has confirmed 4 things:
  1. Your identity
  2. The site of the surgery (e.g. your right hip or your left eye)
  3. The type of surgery (e.g. hip replacement or cataract surgery)
  4. You have read, understand and signed the consent form for the surgery

☐ The site has been marked (usually with a pen or marker)—you can confirm this too

☐ The Anesthesia Team has performed their standard safety checks

☐ The pulse oximeter (described earlier) has been put on and is working properly

☐ Any allergies you have are communicated to the team

☐ Risks of difficulty with managing your airway during the anesthetic are identified (for example, risk of aspirating while asleep)

☐ The risk of significant blood loss is shared and planned for accordingly

---

There is a lot of communication that happens before your surgery even begins. Hopefully, knowing that there are a number of mechanisms in place to keep you safe is reassuring. Some hospitals create modified versions of the Surgical Safety Checklist but the purpose is the same.

Does your hospital use a checklist?

The Anesthetic

It's now time to take the mystery out of anesthesia (some of it, anyway). We'll review the types of anesthetics, how they work, what you'll experience and what goes on while you're under.

---

7 WHO Surgical Safety Checklist and Implementation Manual, 2008, World Health Organization, https://www.who.int/patientsafety/safesurgery/ss_checklist/en/.

How Does Anesthesia Work?

First, they give you a stick to bite on. Then they get out a big rubber mallet...

Very funny, I know (you might actually hear this lame joke in the OR—that's where I got it). Of course, if you required surgery before the discovery of anesthetics in the early 1800s, this might not be far off!

We've come a long way since Dr. William T.G. Morton pioneered the use of ether in 1846—though, this was truly a miracle drug at that time. Fortunately for those having surgery today, anesthesia medications have been developed much further to prevent you from being aware, having pain and moving during an operation.

Let's spend a little time on the types of anesthetics and some little nuggets of information to help you better understand how it's done, starting with everyone's favourite—the IV.

The IV

We touched on the IV a little earlier but let's explore this a little more now.

Most anesthesia medications are given through an intravenous (IV) catheter—nearly everyone gets one. Understandably, this can be a source of anxiety for some people. This next section will help you prepare and know what to expect.

Needles are no fun—fair enough.

That said, the IV *usually* goes in with little difficulty and sometimes local anesthetic is used to make it less painful. Other times, starting an IV can be a challenge... we'll get to that.

The process is straightforward—the clinician takes a large elastic band (called a *tourniquet*) and wraps it around your arm (just tight enough to keep blood from leaving your arm). Blood goes into your arm but can't flow back out past the tourniquet. This engorges your veins with blood, making them larger and easier to see.

Your skin is then cleaned with a disinfectant swab, such as alcohol. You'll probably notice them tapping or slapping the back your hand... oddly enough, this causes the veins to pop up even more. The bigger and easier they are to see, the easier it is to put in the IV.

Next, your skin is stretched slightly to keep the vein stable as the IV catheter is inserted. The needle portion is removed and only the soft plastic catheter remains in your vein—it shouldn't hurt much once it's in (if it hurts a lot, let them know). The catheter is hooked up to IV tubing through which fluid and medications (including most anesthetic drugs) can be given. A dressing secures the catheter in place.

💡 INSIDER TIP

MAKING THE IV EASIER ON YOU

Getting an IV in your hand or arm can be quick and easy… the truth is, it could also be a difficult experience. Here are a few tips for you that could make a big difference:

PREPARING YOUR VEINS:

- Build your muscles. If you are able, resistance training in the weeks prior to your surgery will help build muscle mass. More mass means that more blood flow is required to feed those muscles—this makes those veins start to pop as they grow to move the additional blood flow. If you can, try these: 1) bicep curls, 2) tricep extensions, 3) wrist curls and other grip-strengthening exercises. These will work great (plus, you'll look great too!).

- Stay well hydrated. Drink clear fluids until the cutoff time given to you.

- Stay warm. On the morning of surgery, take the warm blankets that are offered to you and keep your arms tucked under them.

MANAGING DIFFICULT IVs:

- If you've previously experienced a difficult IV insertion, be sure to let the next person know—in particular, let them know where the last person ended up having success! This is also a situation where it is very reasonable to request that a staff clinician attempt the IV, rather than a student. There is a time and place for learning—it doesn't have to be every time.

- Even if you've never had an IV before, if you are in the situation where someone has tried two or three times without success, it is perfectly reasonable to ask if another clinician could provide assistance—this is teamwork and should be well received.

You probably have a pretty good idea already how easy it will be to find your veins. If you have difficulty finding your veins, others will too. If this is the case, make an extra effort to follow through on Preparing Your Veins above. You'll thank yourself.

Special note: There are certain conditions when it's best to avoid starting an IV on a particular arm. For example, people who have had a mastectomy with lymph node removal should ideally have an IV placed on the side opposite to the mastectomy. Also, when the surgery is on a hand or arm, the IV is generally placed on the other side. If any such situation applies to you, communicate this clearly to the person starting the IV. There are certainly exceptions to these examples which makes conversations with your clinical team all the more important in these scenarios.

If the idea of an IV concerns (or scares) you, or if having an IV inserted has been difficult for you in the past, there are ways to help you through the experience. For example, local anesthetic creams can be applied to numb the skin (this is commonly done with kids). Local anesthetic can also be injected with a tiny needle that is much smaller than the IV catheter itself. If the IV is being inserted in the OR, you could be given laughing gas (nitrous oxide) to breathe through a mask. This gas not only helps reduce anxiety, it is also an effective pain reliever—a nice combination for someone anxious about getting an IV. For more on this topic, check out the Insider Tip "Making the IV Easier on You."

The Menu of Anesthesia

Once the IV has been started, the essential monitors have been put on and the "Sign In" checklist has been completed, one of three scenarios will follow depending on the procedure you're having and your anesthesia assessment:

1. Local Anesthesia

Some procedures are performed with a *local anesthetic* to numb or freeze only the small area being worked on. Interestingly, local anesthetics are great at preventing pain signals to the brain but patients often still say that they can feel pressure at the site of surgery. You may have experienced something similar at the dentist—during a tooth filling, for example.

Local anesthetics are used mainly for surgeries that affect a small, superficial part of your body. These medications can be applied topically (such as eye drops) or injected (as with tooth fillings). Examples include everything from removal of skin lesions to eye surgeries to cardiac pacemaker insertions.

Along with this, *sedative medications* may be given to help you feel more relaxed and less aware of the procedure. This technique is also called *conscious* or *procedural sedation*. You can still talk and respond to commands but it is possible that you may have little memory of the situation.

2. Regional Anesthesia

Regional anesthesia prevents pain for large areas of the body. Rather than injecting local anesthetic medications in the specific part of the body being operated on (as with local anesthesia), the medications are instead injected around nerves that go to and from the area/region of your body being worked on.

This causes a loss of sensation to a region of your body (e.g. an arm; your legs). You will commonly be given *sedative medications* for procedures requiring a regional anesthetic to help you stay relaxed. For longer procedures, such as joint replacements, sedation is tremendously helpful in giving you the feeling that time is passing much quicker than it is and taking away the physical discomfort of laying in one position for a long time.

Here are the types of regional anesthetics:

SPINAL ANESTHETIC

- This involves the injection of a small amount of medication around the nerves that supply your lower body.

- A tiny needle is inserted into your lower back (using local anesthesia). Once the tip of the needle is in the right place, anesthetic medication is injected and bathes the lower portion of your spinal cord—this prevents pain signals from your lower body from being sent to your brain. No signal, no pain.

- Spinal anesthetics are used for many surgeries, including knee replacements, hip replacements and Caesarean sections.

EPIDURAL ANESTHETICS

- Rather than just a one-time injection of anesthetic medication as we see with spinal anesthetics, an epidural involves placing a small, flexible catheter just outside the fluid-filled space of the spinal cord. As with spinal anesthetics, it again involves a needle that is inserted into the midline of your back—freezing medications are used here too so it doesn't hurt. You will feel pressure, though.

- Different types of medications can be given continuously through this catheter to give you long-lasting pain relief after surgery, or during labour just ahead of childbirth.

- Epidurals are primarily used for pain relief after surgery, but can sometimes be used for the surgery itself. You might be aware that women in labour often benefit from epidurals to help with pain control. There are many other operations that benefit from an epidurals too, particularly major surgeries on the chest and abdomen.

PERIPHERAL NERVE BLOCK

- This is a clever type of pain control for surgery. Let's say you're having surgery on your hand. There are many small nerves that supply your hand and it would be challenging to freeze them all with local anesthetics. If you move up to your shoulder, there are only a few larger nerves that take care of your whole arm and hand.

- In fact, these larger nerves can been seen using ultrasound—pretty cool. While looking at them under ultrasound, anesthetic medications can be injected all around them. So now, no pain information coming from the hand during surgery can reach the brain—no signal, no pain!

- Surgery on the arm and hand are great candidates for a peripheral nerve block. So are certain foot surgeries and sometimes even shoulder surgery. This can also be a great way to control pain after surgery using catheters similar to the epidural.

Some Thoughts for You Regarding Local & Regional Anesthesia

A member of your Anesthesia Team will decide with you if local or regional anesthesia is appropriate for you. There are definitely some benefits over having a general anesthetic, when appropriate. Let's talk about the advantages.

First of all, sedative medications used in anesthesia work *really* well! Many people who have received sedation for a procedure end up remembering very little of the surgery. Others will remember everything, most recalling that they were fairly relaxed throughout the whole procedure. No fear, no stress. The drugs work well and we know how to use them.

Secondly, your recovery from a procedure is often much faster when you receive sedation rather than a general anesthetic. You're also less likely to have nausea and vomiting too—a pretty common side effect of a general anesthetic.

There are risks associated with whatever route you take. There are just too many variations to cover all of the possible risks here—that's what your OR team assesses for with every patient. Just know that all of the information on your Ready for My Surgery Checklist, along with all of the assessments and tests you receive, weigh into the final determination of your individual risks for any procedure.

3. **General Anesthesia**

For many surgeries, a local or regional anesthetic just isn't an option. So, off to sleep you go.

By now, I'm sure you've gathered that a general anesthetic involves more than just "putting you to sleep," though that is part of it.

Let's break this thing down a little.

A general anesthetic is designed to prevent you from having awareness or pain during surgery. There are three main parts or phases to this anesthetic:

💡 INSIDER TIP

ABOUT SEDATION
Calm and relaxed versus stressed and anxious

This is the general goal of giving sedative medication to a patient for a procedure. Just because a general anesthetic isn't required doesn't mean the patient isn't still nervous—in fact, many people get more anxious when they find out they'll be awake for the whole thing!

Here's the deal—because you're awake, you can talk. Because you can talk, you can communicate how you feel. You have the ability to work with your anesthesia care provider to tailor the anesthetic to your needs to a large degree.

Different scenarios call for different "depths" of sedation. Your anesthesiologist or anesthesia assistant will know how to manage this. Just remember, sedation (even deep sedation—meaning, you are heavily sedated) is different than a general anesthetic. You'll be aware. You may be happy as a lark, but you should expect to have some awareness and recollection of the situation.

- **First, you are "put to sleep"—the *Induction Phase of Anesthesia***
  - Think of this phase like you're taking off in an airplane—lots of preparation, activity and change

- **Next, you are kept asleep during the surgery—the *Maintenance Phase of Anesthesia***
  - Now, you're at your cruising altitude—steady and stable is the goal

- **Lastly, you are awakened—the *Emergence Phase of Anesthesia***
  - The plane lands—another busy time with lots of activity

How Does a General Anesthetic Work?
A specific combination of medications given at just the right time and just the right dose will take you to that happy place. The way anesthesia professionals look at it, there are three main parts to this drug regimen which is called the Triad of Anesthesia (cool name). Here's the triad:

1. Hypnosis (the *unconsciousness* part)
3. Analgesia (the *pain control* part)
4. Muscle Relaxation (the *preventing you from moving during surgery* part)

These three things are accomplished with drugs that have been developed and refined over time to make anesthetics safe and effective. The drug type, dose and timing are determined by taking the following into consideration:

- Your physiology (how your body works, including your health issues)

- The medications you take

- Your age, weight and gender

- The anesthetic medications that were chosen for you

- The other medications you need (e.g. fluids, antibiotics, drugs to prevent nausea after surgery, drugs to treat your blood pressure, etc.)

- The impact of surgery on your physiology (e.g. blood loss, pain/stimulation, effects on organ function, etc.)

- Your response to the medications you were given (not everyone reacts the same way)

Sounds like a lot more than putting you to sleep! And so it is. All of these factors are monitored, analyzed and taken into consideration during your anesthetic. This guides the anesthesiologist to continuously fine tune the anesthetic to meet your individual needs.

During a flight things can change quickly—particularly during take-off and landing. Even at cruising altitude you can run into turbulence. Anesthesia practice is often compared to aviation, particularly as it relates to checklists, safety and vigilance. Your Anesthesia Team must be vigilant in monitoring, identifying and treating the turbulence that can arise during your ride through surgery and anesthesia. This is a continuous process extending before, during and after your surgery (collectively called the *perioperative period*—literally, the time surrounding the operation).

Let's Go to Sleep

You know it's coming when the mask is heading for your face... Don't worry, it's just oxygen. And getting a little oxygen before a general anesthetic is a really good idea. This extra O_2 (oxygen's chemical name) gives the anesthetist time to "secure your airway" once you're asleep. If having a mask placed over your face makes you feel claustrophobic, ask to hold the mask yourself. Some people find this to be very helpful.

After breathing through this mask for a few minutes, the anesthetic drugs will begin flowing through the IV. The most common anesthetic used today for the induction of anesthesia is called propofol—it's uniquely white in colour and it works fast! One downside is that it often stings when it's injected.

One strange thing about having an anesthetic is your perception of time. When you wake up, you'll feel as if no time has passed. This can be a bit disorienting, particularly when you wake up in a place different from where you went to sleep (the Post-Anesthetic Care Unit (PACU), for example).

What Actually Happens While I'm Asleep?

Once you are asleep (Maintenance Phase), the team will run through the next part of the WHO checklist before beginning the surgery.

This is called the "Time Out":

TIME OUT—BEFORE SURGERY BEGINS[8]

- ☐ Each person in the Operating Room introduces themselves by name and role (in large hospitals, team members can change regularly)
- ☐ The patient's name, site of surgery and type of surgery are confirmed once again
- ☐ Confirmation that antibiotics have been given, if applicable
- ☐ The surgeon, anesthesiologist and nurse take turns communicating information critical to the surgery as well as any concerns
- ☐ Essential imaging (such as x-rays, CT scans or MRIs) is displayed, if applicable

---

You will then be positioned carefully and secured to the OR table to keep you in that position. Your skin will be cleaned using an antiseptic solution where the surgery will take place. Sterile drapes (sheets) cover all of you except the area that the surgeons need to access. The equipment and instruments needed for surgery are brought into place.

It's pretty easy to get really cold in the OR—you may notice that the OR is quite cold when you walk in. Being cold during surgery can delay your recovery and increase your risk of getting an infection, amongst other problems. To prevent your body temperature from dropping (called *hypothermia*), warming blankets are used—some you lay on, some lay on you.

During all of this, your anesthesiologist is busy monitoring your vital signs and administering fluids and various medications, including antibiotics. Before surgery begins, the surgeon will ask the anesthesiologist if it is okay to start. This is an important piece of teamwork that adds to the safety of the operation.

Family & Friends—Let's Look After Them Too

For family and friends, there will be a space in the hospital for them to wait while the surgery is underway. Updates will typically be provided at the end of surgery.

---

8 WHO Surgical Safety Checklist and Implementation Manual, 2008, World Health Organization, https://www.who.int/patientsafety/safesurgery/ss_checklist/en/.

During longer surgeries, intermittent updates may be given so that your friends and family can have a sense of how it is going.

Rather than just sit and wait, encourage your loved ones to walk, read, eat and drink. This will help the time go by more quickly and could reduce any anxiety they may be feeling.

Finished! Surgery Is Over

A few important things happen in the OR at the end of surgery:

- The post-surgical checklist, called the "Sign Out," is performed to ensure the outcome of the surgery is well documented, any issues are addressed and your recovery plan is discussed:

SIGN OUT—BEFORE THE PATIENT LEAVES THE OPERATING ROOM[9]

☐ The nurse communicates:

1. The name of the surgery that was entered into the patient chart
2. The final count of all items matches the count at the beginning
3. Any specimens (such as a tissue sample) are properly labelled
4. If any equipment issues need to be addressed

☐ The surgeon, anesthesiologist and nurse review the immediate plan for the patient's recovery

☐ Pain medications are given and adjusted to control the pain associated with your surgery

☐ Your breathing, blood pressure, heart rate, oxygen saturation and other vital signs are carefully monitored and can be treated, if necessary

☐ Your anesthetic is reversed (i.e. Emergence Phase—the plane lands)

Emergence—Some Details About How You Wake Up

The drugs keeping you sedated or asleep are generally stopped at the end of surgery while you are still in the Operating Room. All drugs have an expected duration of action (i.e. the length of time they will have an effect on your body). This allows your emergence to be timed with the end of surgery. You will be monitored very closely during this time.

---

9   WHO Surgical Safety Checklist and Implementation Manual, 2008, World Health Organization, https://www.who.int/patientsafety/safesurgery/ss_checklist/en/.

If your anesthetic requires that you have an artificial airway inserted, the removal of this airway is a special procedure, called *extubation*. This is often performed in the OR once you are awake enough to protect your own airway (i.e. prevent yourself from aspirating). More on this shortly.

For some people, the "waking up" is a source of anxiety. If the anticipation of this or any other part of the process is causing you to feel nervous, be sure to ask about this when you speak with the anesthesiologist, AA or CRNA.

Post-Anesthetic Care Unit

After your surgery has finished, you'll leave the OR and be taken to another area to recover—this space is generally called the Post-Anesthetic Care Unit, or PACU for short. It's typically a large, open room with beds that are easy to see for the nursing staff. It's a busy spot with patients always coming and going.

If the anesthetic was the flight (take-off, cruising and landing), the PACU is the baggage claim. The excitement is over and sometimes you end up hanging around here while you wait for your bags.

What can you expect here? The PACU is staffed by a team of nurses that work with your anesthesia and surgical teams to:

- Monitor your recovery from the anesthetic
- Assess and treat your pain and nausea
- Assess the site of surgery and monitor for any issues, such as bleeding
- Arrange for tests that are needed after surgery, such as x-rays or ultrasound
- Access specialty support, such as Respiratory Therapists for intensive breathing support
- Talk to you, help you get oriented after your anesthetic and answer your questions
- Begin some early recovery routines with you, such as deep breathing exercises
- Support your transition to the Hospital Ward or home
- In the spirit of air travel, consider the above as all of the bags that need to be claimed before you can move on!

Waking Up in the PACU

Most of the time, your anesthetic will be reversed in the OR and you will be awake (to some degree) when you arrive in the PACU. For various reasons, you may remain under anesthesia in the PACU for a short time. If this is the case, your anesthetic will be reversed in the PACU—the process is essentially the same as it would be in the OR.

A common concern of those having an anesthetic is the unpredictable behaviour that can occur as they wake up. Some people feel worried that they may say something unintended or inappropriate. While it's true that your brain may not be firing on all cylinders at first, the PACU staff are quite used to dealing with this and are there to help you through this transition.

Your Memory After Anesthesia

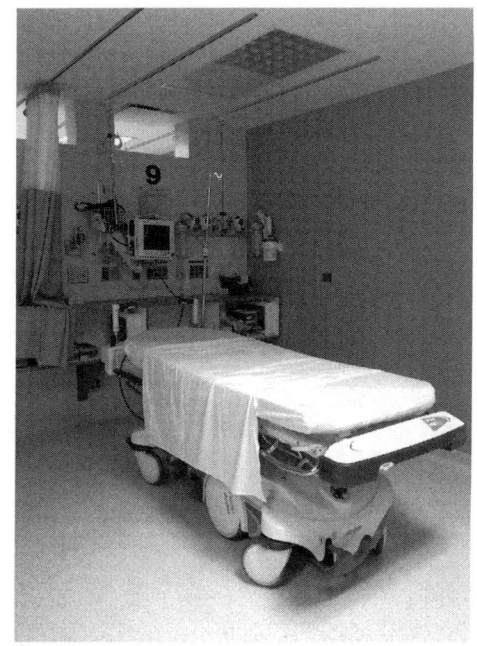

You'll certainly want to know how your operation went, but I'd like to offer this advice—don't feel compelled to ask about the details just after you've woken up. Why? Your memory.

Your short-term memory can be affected by the lingering anesthetics circulating in your bloodstream. You may ask lots of questions and get lots of answers but a short time later, you may remember none of it! The staff in the PACU are quite used to this.

You shouldn't be concerned about this common side effect; it'll wear off as the medications do. If you have lingering issues with your memory, let your doctor know.

Give yourself a chance to recover from the anesthetic and rest before asking too many questions. Was the outcome of the surgery as you and your surgeon had planned? This much you'll want to know—the details can come later.

Sore Throat After Anesthesia

Another common complaint after an anesthetic is a sore throat. With general anesthetics, an artificial airway is used to help support your breathing—this is most often the cause of the sore throat. To give you a sense of what these are, here's a brief description of the two main types:

ENDOTRACHEAL TUBES (ETT)
- These are plastic tubes that are inserted through your mouth or nose, ending up in your trachea (commonly called your windpipe—a much more descriptive term... kind of funny too).

- The tip sits just below your vocal cords (inside your "Adam's Apple"... the medical word for this is *larynx*).

- A small balloon encircles the ETT just before its tip. Inflating this balloon helps prevent fluid or stomach contents from going into your lungs—a good thing! It also makes sure the air pushed into your lungs by the breathing machine (i.e. mechanical ventilator—it's part of the anesthesia machine) doesn't leak out.

- If you have a sore throat after surgery, the ETT and the process of its insertion (called *endotracheal intubation*) is usually the culprit.

SUPRALARYNGEAL AIRWAY/LARYNGEAL MASK AIRWAY (LMA)
- This is a very clever device invented by a doctor named Archie Brain in 1988—great name.

- It has a formed, inflatable ring that when placed in the back of the throat, creates a sealed pathway for air to flow in and out of the lungs.

- There are now a number of variations of this device on the market. They are known to be easier to place and create less sore throats than an ETT.[10]

Your anesthesiologist will be familiar with both types of artificial airways and will select the best one for you based on your particular needs.

When the anesthetic medications wear off and you begin to wake up, you may find yourself coughing and/or becoming aware of an uncomfortable sensation in your throat. Now you know what it is! *You may remember this part.* Don't be concerned if you do—you need to be conscious enough to protect your airway before the ETT/LMA is removed. It doesn't hurt, it's just uncomfortable.

Feeling Sick
General anesthesia can also make you feel sick to your stomach. Unfortunately, it can lead to vomiting too. This is a known side effect of general anesthetics called

---

[10] Kariem El-Boghdadly et al., "Postoperative Sore Throat: A Systematic Review." *Anaesthesia* (2016), https://onlinelibrary.wiley.com/doi/10.1111/anae.13438.

post-operative nausea and vomiting (PONV). It's an unpleasant side effect but there are a number of medications to treat this when it occurs.

Important Note: If you've previously had nausea and vomiting after surgery, be sure to *tell your anesthesia care provider.* There are a number of ways to prevent it if they know.

Pain Control

How you experience pain could be quite different than another person that has had the same operation. Because of this, standard ways of assessing pain have been developed so that each person can be treated according to their unique experience.

This particular aspect of your care is one that requires strong communication between you and your healthcare providers. *There is no need to be stoic and just deal with the pain.* In fact, poor pain control can actually impair your recovery. Be as accurate as you can with how you rate your pain and communicate this to your healthcare team.

One of the great aspects of modern medicine is our access to an arsenal of very effective pain medications. Your healthcare team will use these as required to keep you as comfortable as possible.

A NOTE ON CHRONIC PAIN: Chronic pain is commonly defined as pain that has lasted more than three months. It's a pretty complex topic—if it applies to you, you'll probably have an appreciation for how your needs for pain control may be different during and after surgery.

In particular, if you take narcotic/opioid medications regularly, such as fentanyl, it is important that the anesthesiologist and surgeon understand exactly what you take and why. If you see a pain specialist, ask for a note that describes your chronic pain history and your treatment regimen. This will help the hospital team best plan to address your specific requirements.

The PACU will probably be the first place you're asked to rate your pain. A standard "pain scale" is used to help you communicate this to your nurse and others involved in your care. Before you leave the PACU, your pain medications will be adjusted so that your pain is well controlled.

Your surgery and anesthetic are now behind you. From here, it's all about your recovery. Sometimes, the biggest challenges and surprises have yet to come. Let's walk through your recovery and have you as prepared for this as you were for the surgery itself.

4

RECOVERING FROM SURGERY

PURPOSE OF THIS CHAPTER
To give you the tools to stay safe, expect the unexpected and optimize your recovery so you can get back to doing what you do as quickly as possible.

KEY THINGS WE'LL COVER
- Recovering in hospital—your role and expectations
- The Hospital Ward
- People you may work with after surgery
- First steps to start your recovery on the right path
- Keeping comfortable—managing your pain
- Avoiding infection—managing your wound
- The Intensive Care Unit—special care for special situations
- Recovering at home—preparing you for when the health-care professionals are no longer immediately available to answer your questions
- Stories from people who have been in your shoes—we'll learn from their experiences

HOW DO YOU think you might feel after surgery?

Groggy? Hazy? Maybe a little nauseous? If any of these crossed your mind, you're not far off.

General anesthetics, in general... take time to recover from and you may not feel too well in the first few hours afterward.

Following *minor* surgery, you may quickly get back to feeling and looking yourself. For *major* surgery, how you look and feel can vary dramatically.

No doubt about it—some surgeries are harder on you than others. The location, type of incision and invasiveness of a surgery are factors that influence this. The amount of pain associated with surgery can vary and the medications taken to treat this pain have their own potential side effects.

Some operations can significantly impact one's appearance, such as head and neck surgery or amputation. Surgeries that alter a person's appearance can have profound psychological and social implications that are beyond the scope of this book. If this topic applies to you, having a plan for support and counselling before and after surgery are as important as the preparation this book offers—talk to your surgeon about their recommendations.

Consider this: The time it will take for you to recover from surgery will likely be *much longer* than the operation itself. You may be on your own for much of the recovery too, with reduced access to doctors and other healthcare professionals once you go home.

That said, you've prepared well for the day of surgery. Let's now do the same for your recovery.

Space to Recover

As you've learned, the PACU is the place where much of your anesthetic will wear off. The goal here is to make sure that you are recovering well from the anesthetic and your pain is controlled before moving to your next destination. This next destination will be:

- **The Hospital Ward**—If you are spending one or more nights in hospital
- **The Intensive Care Unit (ICU)**—If you need special care after your surgery
- **Home**—If you're having day surgery

Let's start with your recovery in hospital. We'll finish off the chapter by talking about going home.

Recovery in the Hospital Ward

You & Your Healthcare Team

Part of the preparation you've already done will help you after surgery as well. In your Ready for My Surgery Checklist, you'll have written down a number of things that will help you understand *what to expect*.

The expected length of your recovery, challenges you may face and things you can do to optimize your recovery are all great to know; but there's more:

What should your expectations be of the healthcare team while you're in hospital?

There's an approach called Patient-Centred Care (PCC) that many healthcare institutions have embraced. Sounds good, right? Putting you at the centre of your healthcare? It is good. The culture within many hospitals has shifted toward this philosophy of patient care in recent years.

It's not just a one-sided activity, though. On one hand, it takes the healthcare provider to engage in conversation with you as a patient about all aspects of your care. On the other hand, a patient must feel empowered to engage these professionals on level ground. *Not a hierarchy*—professionals know their craft but they don't know you, not to the degree where they can assume to know what is important to you.

What is important to you needs to be important to all. This doesn't mean you always get what you want—it means that you'll collaborate to decide on a plan for your care.

Being treated as an individual is important for many reasons:

- Your treatments are tailored to *your* needs and preferences
- Your personal goals and needs are understood, allowing them to be supported (for example, you may find comfort in speaking with someone from spiritual care while you're in hospital—if this is known, it's much more likely to happen)
- You feel like a person, not just another patient
- Your experience is more likely to be positive and provide you needed motivation during your early recovery
- A positive experience can (and hopefully will) lead to positive feedback to healthcare providers, as well as to the hospital itself, which reinforces this practice (we'll talk about giving feedback in the next chapter)

Is there more? For sure, but I'll let someone else offer a perspective now—someone who's been in your shoes.

In Your Shoes

PATRICIA'S STORY

Patricia told me some interesting things about her experience of having surgery. We talked a lot while I was writing this book. She was very honest and thoughtful as she usually is. I should mention, Patricia is my mother-in-law and she refers to me as her favorite son-in-law (I'm quite okay with that, despite being her only son-in-law).

She's had a few surgeries over the years and she is a courageous cancer survivor. The story she shared with me was related to her most recent surgery—a total hip replacement. Here are some tips, from her to you:

BEFORE SURGERY:
- Acceptance really helped make the experience less stressful—she embraced the fact that the surgery could help her and was grateful that she could have the operation. This kept her from unnecessary (and unhelpful) worry.
- After sharing the fact that she was scheduled for surgery with a few people, she stopped. It seems that well-intentioned friends sometimes feel compelled

to share troubling stories of surgeries that didn't go well for one reason or another. She didn't find this particularly helpful (surprise!). So, consider who you share this with—stick with people who will keep your best interests in mind and will be supportive and positive.

AFTER SURGERY:

In hospital:
- Her saving grace was music—she brought her favourite music and earphones from home and used it often. It was relaxing and gave her a warm distraction from the busy Hospital Ward activities surrounding her. Maybe this could help you too?

At home:
- She found it took a good couple weeks to really start feeling herself again
- She found that she wanted more time alone during those first couple weeks
- Regular, short visits and check-ins by friends and family helped a lot

Patricia also had a couple of challenges during her recovery that we can learn from.

The first was the lack of choice she felt when it came time for her to take pain medications on the ward. The situation wasn't uncommon—her nurse brought pain medications to her bedside and asked her to take them. The issue for Patricia was that she wasn't having any pain. She told this to the nurse but she was told that she should still take them. (Remember the section earlier about pain? If you wait too long to take pain medication, it can be hard to get the pain under control again.) So she took them.

Patricia knew that opioid medications (such as morphine and the like) didn't agree with her. Unfortunately, the nausea and vomiting that she subsequently experienced was very unpleasant and left her frustrated that she ended up taking medications that she didn't really want to.

Do you think anything could have been improved in this exchange between the patient and healthcare provider?

Patricia didn't even know she was prescribed a standard dose of narcotics until she was presented with them. Would she have felt more in control and more comfortable if this had been discussed with her ahead of time? She may have still needed these medications (and still felt sick after) but how she felt about the situation could have been entirely different. This is a goal of patient engagement and Patient-Centred Care (PCC).

Being part of the plan helps people get on board with it.

Patricia's second issue was also related to prescription medications. Once home, she started a new medication that, as a side effect, caused her hands to swell quite a bit. Since it was the only new medication she was taking, she figured that it was the cause and decided to just stop taking it.

Should she have? Did she really know why she was taking that medication?

These aren't questions we need to answer here. The point is, if you are having an issue such as this, will you know what to do? Maybe not... this is the benefit of having a plan. Knowing whom to contact for questions and knowing when to seek immediate care (such as going to the Emergency Room) is invaluable when you're on your own at home and an issue arises. Your Ready for My Surgery Checklist will be the foundation of this plan.

Patricia had an excellent recovery from her hip replacement. She was diligent in doing her physiotherapy and other rehabilitation activities. Good thing too—she's got a couple of busy grandchildren that keep her hopping!

Thanks for sharing, Patricia.

***

The Hospital Ward

A Hospital Ward is a section of a hospital dedicated to providing care to inpatients (patients staying one or more nights). For you, this will be a Surgical Ward. Rooms on Hospital Wards often support multiple patients, though private rooms are generally available as well (some insurance policies cover private rooms).

I've been introducing you to the people you're likely to meet along the way. Not surprisingly, there are a few more to add to the list that will support your recovery. I'll keep it brief but will direct you to more information should you be interested in reading more.

People on the Ward

There's a team of healthcare providers that will routinely monitor your recovery and keep you on track so that your discharge from hospital will be on time.

Here are the usual suspects:

DOCTORS OF ALL SORTS
- In addition to your surgeon, there's a long list of different specialties in medicine and it's possible that you may find yourself in need of the services of one of them—some examples are:

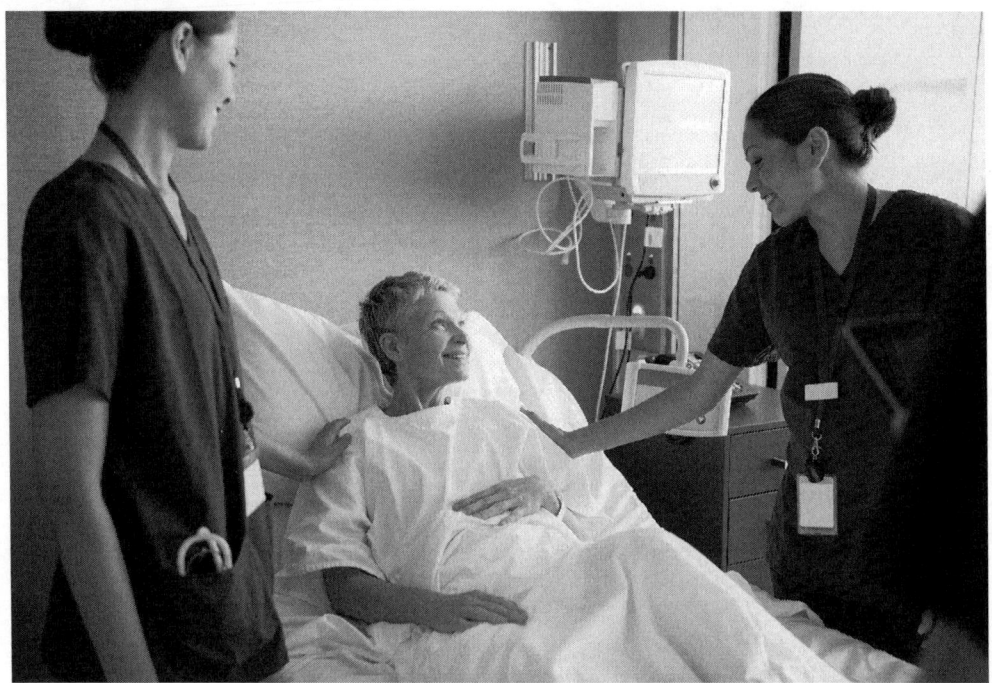

- Respirologists (lung specialists—also known as pulmonologists)
- Cardiologists (heart specialists)
- Neurologists (brain and nervous system specialists)

• If so (and you're feeling up to it), be curious and ask them about their role and how they hope to support your recovery

• If you'd like to know more about different medical specialties, I'd encourage you to visit the website of the medical association for your country (e.g. American Medical Association at www.ama-assn.org or Canadian Medical Association at www.cma.ca)

PHYSIOTHERAPISTS (PT) & PHYSIOTHERAPIST ASSISTANTS (PTA)
- These folks will support your physical rehabilitation after surgery to optimize recovery of your mobility and physical functioning (they'll teach you the keys to a great physical recovery).

- Physiotherapists are called Physical Therapists in the US

OCCUPATIONAL THERAPISTS (OT) & OCCUPATIONAL THERAPIST ASSISTANTS (OTA)

- These are the people who will help enable you to do whatever activities that you need to do throughout your day. There will be many things you won't be able to do as usual after surgery and your OT will give you the tools to do them. Even common things like getting dressed, bathing and moving around your home can pose a challenge early on.

REGISTERED RESPIRATORY THERAPISTS (RT)

- We've covered RTs already but as a reminder, these are specialists in most everything related to breathing. Most people don't see an RT after surgery but if you're having an immediate issue that is affecting your breathing, they'll be there to look after you.

REGISTERED NURSES (RN)

- Nurses on the Hospital Ward are the highly-skilled backbone of the ward. They often carry heavy workloads and heavy responsibility to ensure each patient in their care is not only recovering well but also able to participate fully in their care—a tall order indeed.

REGISTERED PRACTICAL NURSES (RPN)

- Another important professional member of the nursing team in most wards—direct patient care is their specialty.

PHARMACISTS

- Much like your local pharmacist, a hospital pharmacist looks after your medications. This is an important and often complicated task that takes into account your medical history, mix of medications, allergies and surgery-specific medication needs.

PHYSICIAN ASSISTANTS (PA)

- Physician Assistants are relatively new to the Canadian public healthcare system, though the Canadian military have had PAs since the 1980s. This profession has been around even longer in the US. Considered physician extenders, they have a valuable role of increasing the capacity of the healthcare system to deliver care under the supervision of a physician. You may see them in many different fields, including primary and emergency care.

REGISTERED DIETICIANS
- These professionals use their knowledge of your body's metabolism during healing to make sure you're getting the type of nutrition you need to help with your recovery.

NURSE PRACTITIONERS (NP)
- These are RNs that have pursued additional university training and function in a variety of roles. For example, pain management after surgery can be complex. Many hospitals have a team called the Acute Pain Service to support these patients—Nurse Practitioners are generally key members of this team.

SOCIAL WORKERS
- Linking you and your family with the healthcare team or with community resources in a holistic way are just a couple of ways that Social Workers facilitate getting you the care you need. They can also be a wonderful resource should you be struggling with any personal issues during your hospital stay.

SPEECH-LANGUAGE PATHOLOGISTS (SLP)
- These smart folks are specialized in helping people with problems related to, well... speech and language. They are experts in communication. They are also specialists in swallowing and feeding/eating issues—a problem that presents itself in the hospital following certain surgeries.

SPIRITUAL CARE
- In most hospitals, a Chaplain will be part of the healthcare team and acts to support your spiritual and religious needs.

OTHER HOSPITAL STAFF
- There are other staff that you may meet along the way, such as attendants, volunteers and other professionals I didn't mention. They all play an important role in creating a healthcare environment that is caring, effective and efficient.

More Information on Healthcare Professionals
To get more information on any healthcare profession, there are two main places to go:

Professional Associations
- The role of these organizations is to advocate for the profession itself
- To find one, do an internet search using the following keywords:
    1. Name of the profession
    1. "association" or "society"
    2. Country or region (state, province) you are interested in
- Here's an example:
    - In Google, I entered the keywords "respiratory therapy association canada"—here are my results:

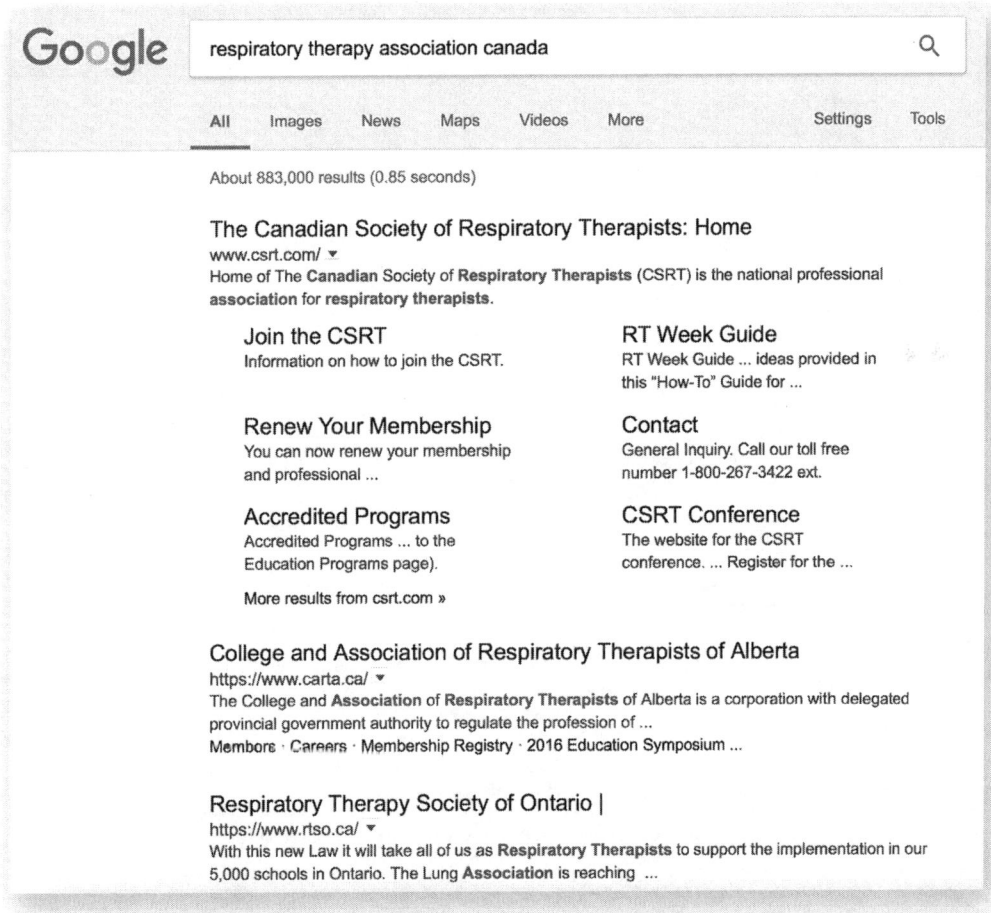

Google and the Google logo are registered trademarks of Google Inc., used with permission.

Professional Regulatory Colleges

- These organizations have a primary mandate to protect the public (that's you) by ensuring consistent and competent practice by their members.

- Each regulated health profession will have its own College. This is the place to go should you have any questions or concerns about a healthcare profession or one of its members.

- To find a profession's College, use keywords
  1. Name of the profession (e.g. "respiratory therapy")
  3. "regulatory body"
  4. Country or region (state, province) you are interested in

- Here's an example:
  - In Google, I entered the keywords "respiratory therapy regulatory body ontario"—here are my results:

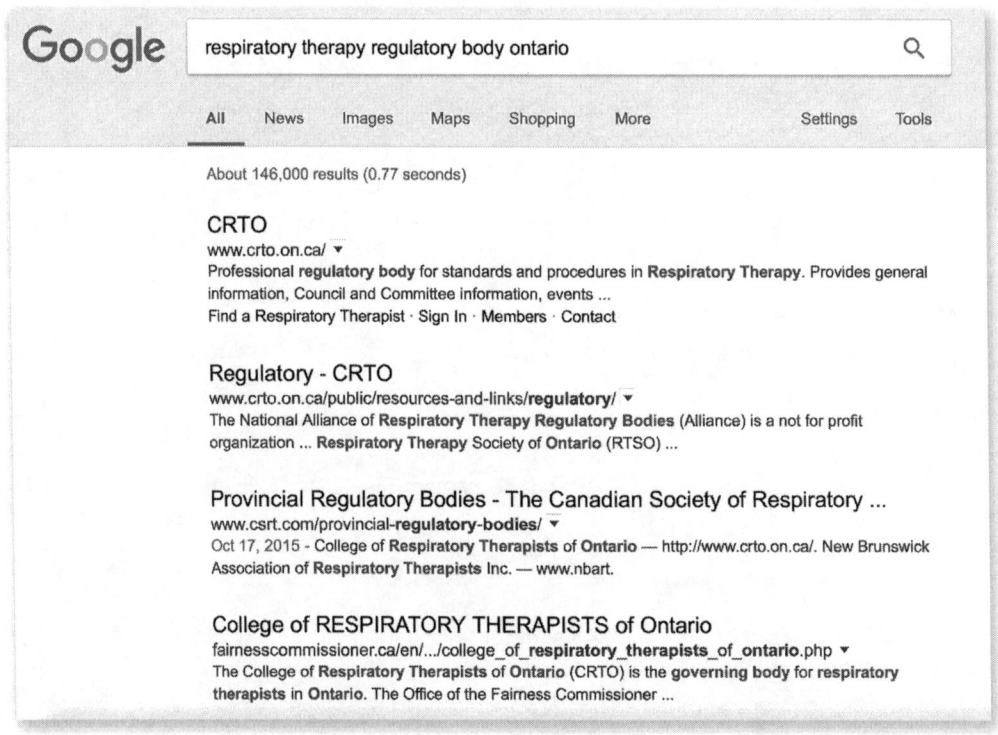

Google and the Google logo are registered trademarks of Google Inc., used with permission.

Your Job on the Ward
Now your work begins...
Much more may be required of you after surgery than during your preparation. You'll be asked lots of questions and will be given lots of instructions and things to do (e.g. deep breathing, therapy exercises, etc.). It's fair to say that you'll have many, although short, exchanges with many different people. Let's cover the main things you'll need to do to keep your recovery on track.

Knowing the Plan
The nursing staff are the constant on the ward, the foundation. It's hard to imagine a nurse on the ward that isn't busy! They've got a lot of tasks to manage with a lot of patients—this requires them to be efficient. Doctors generally visit you briefly once a day and other professionals join in your care as needed. Based on the description of the professionals listed above, you should have a good idea of when that would be.

The time spent with you by each person may be short and fast. If you know your plan for recovery, it'll be easier for you to work together with them.

There will be a daily plan for your recovery. If you are able, you should be participating in its development. Discussing the plan and asking questions about it will help you understand what will happen and what is expected of you.

Do I *really* need to know the plan? They've got it under control, right?

Well, maybe.

Can your healthcare team really have the best plan for you if you're not involved? Is your plan specific to *you* or just "patients like you"?

Hospitals dedicated to patient engagement know that your participation with, and understanding of, your care plan improves patient safety and satisfaction. If your hospital provided you with or recommended this book, it is highly likely that this is a goal of that organization.

Let's move on to the practical things that will help you with your recovery.

Get Moving
Exercise after surgery prevents physical deconditioning (losing muscle). If you can, get out of bed. If you can't get out of bed, you may still be able to do some exercise. Here are a few staple exercises—ask your healthcare team if you can do these:

1. **Deep Breathing Exercises (Get Those Alveoli Open and Filled with Air!)**
You may be asked to do some deep breathing (they may give you a device to breathe into that gives deep breathing a fancy name—*incentive spirometry*). This is done

> **🔍 INTERESTING FACT**
>
> *Alveoli* are tiny, air-filled spaces that create a honeycomb-like interconnected network at the end of your smallest airways. When you breathe in, this is where the air ends up. Tiny blood vessels (called *capillaries*) line these alveoli. This is where the magic of *respiration* (gas exchange) happens. Oxygen moves from the alveoli into your blood and carbon dioxide moves from your blood into the alveoli. When you breathe in and out, you are adding more oxygen to the alveoli and clearing the carbon dioxide—cool stuff!

to help prevent lung infections by keeping your lungs open and stable. If you can't breathe deeply because of pain, work with your hospital team to get this pain under control. The consequences of taking only shallow breaths for a prolonged period of time aren't good—collapse of your smallest airways and alveoli (see sidebar) can occur and lead to the need for additional oxygen, as well as put you at risk for developing pneumonia.

2. Exercise (Get Your Blood Flowing!)

Lying around in bed after surgery will put you at higher risk of blood clots forming in your legs—this can actually be life threatening… So, it's worth avoiding.

If you can, moving and exercising your legs is quite helpful in preventing blood clots. Beyond clotting issues, building your strength back after surgery should be a goal for everyone.

As mentioned already, get out of bed if and when you can—the sooner the better. Here are some simple exercises for you to do when you are in bed (be sure to run these by your nurse/surgeon/physiotherapist before you start—some surgeries will have restrictions on what you can do):

- Flex and straighten your legs at the knee, tighten and relax your upper leg muscles (quadriceps and hamstrings)

- Rotate and flex your ankles, then point your toes, tighten and relax your calf muscles

- Tense, then relax the muscles from your feet to your head—get blood moving! *Did you know that blood flow through your veins relies heavily on your muscles contracting and squeezing the veins within them?*

- Stretch—you'll want to ask what types of stretching are okay, this will depend on the type of surgery you've had. This is an important part of any exercise routine.

What if these types of exercise are difficult or just aren't possible? There are other ways to prevent clots from forming and these may be used for your surgery. To prepare you, here are a couple therapies that are used:

- Pressure stockings—you may be prescribed these if you are at high risk for clots, these will help prevent blood from pooling in your legs

- Blood thinners—these medications are used to prevent clotting from happening in the first place. A commonly used medication, called heparin, is given through an injection just under the skin (it's a really tiny needle but it can sting)

Important note: If you are having injections of blood thinners, don't be surprised if you see bruising around the area of injection—you should certainly point it out to your nurse, but this bruising is common.

Eating Well

On the ward, your nurse will perform an assessment of your medical status. Part of that assessment will determine what liquids and solid foods you are ready for. Hopefully, you're ready to eat! If you are, you should—this is part of most Enhanced Recovery After Surgery (ERAS) protocols (we touched on this in Chapter 1). You will have been fasting for a while by this point...

If you have a feeding tube after surgery, that too will be assessed and your nutrition will be looked after accordingly (feeding tubes are pretty common and generally temporary—don't be alarmed if your surgery calls for one, but you should discuss this in some detail with your surgeon if it is part of the plan).

Physical exercise is often a great motivator to help you choose healthy foods. Your pre-surgery exercise routine will help motivate you to eat well and will guide your food choices throughout your recovery. Building lean muscle before your operation is thought to be helpful for recovery because the "stress response" your body has in response to surgery can quickly reduce your lean muscle mass.[1] This *stress response* really messes with both your hormones and your metabolism... Being strong, well-nourished and hydrated can go a long way to lessening the impact this has.

Comforts of Home

While you're in hospital, your food choices may be quite limited. If you have any food allergies, your choices can be even more limited. I'm sure you've heard that hospital food generally doesn't live up to mom's home cooking; although, some hospitals are working hard to improve this.

---

1 Francesco Carli, "Physiologic Considerations of Enhanced Recovery After Surgery (ERAS) Programs: Implications of the Stress Response." *Canadian Journal of Anesthesia* (2015), https://doi.org/10.1007/s12630-014-0264-0.

Familiar foods from home can be nourishing for the body and soul when you're feeling rough after an operation. Speak to your nurse and dietician about what foods can be brought into the hospital, as well as what foods would best serve you during your recovery (e.g. protein, healthy fats, etc.).

Skin Care

Lying in bed can be hard on your skin. Certain parts of your body take more of your weight than others. Prolonged pressure in these areas can lead to something called *pressure sores* (also known as *bed sores*).

Changing positions and getting out of bed regularly (if you can) is helpful to prevent this type of skin breakdown. Pressure sores can become a big problem if left unattended (especially for people with diabetes) and can end up causing a deeper wound (called an *ulcer*).

So, be diligent in checking your skin (or having someone else check), particularly if you are confined to a bed or wheelchair for an extended period of time.

Check the following usual areas for redness (typically they are bony places):

IF LYING IN BED FOR AN EXTENDED PERIOD:
- Back of your head
- Ears
- Shoulder blades
- Tailbone and hips
- Ankles and heels

IF YOU ARE IN A WHEELCHAIR FOR AN EXTENDED PERIOD:
- Back of your arms and legs
- Tailbone, hips and buttocks
- Shoulder blades and along your spine

Looking After Your Incision

You will be taught how to look after your *incision* (the cut made through your skin for surgery—also called a *surgical wound*) before you go home. Pay attention to how your nurse cares for your wound while you're still in the hospital so you can do the same once you're home.

Here are a few tips for looking after your surgical wound:

- Wash your hands well before changing your dressing/bandage
- Wet the dressing a little if it's stuck to the wound

- Wet a clean gauze with saline (salt water) or mild soapy water to clean the wound—ask your nurse or doctor what they recommend
- Don't put any lotions or creams on the wound unless you've been told to
- Always put on a clean dressing (ya, putting on the old one would just be gross)
- Wash your hands again after you're done

HERE ARE THE COMMON WAYS AN INCISION CAN BE CLOSED:
- Stitches
- Staples
- Surgical skin glue
- Small adhesive tape strips

SIGNS YOUR INCISION NEEDS INSPECTION (BY SOMEONE OTHER THAN YOU):
- It's becoming more red or painful
- It's becoming more swollen
- It starts bleeding or the wound opens
- It starts to smell bad or has pus discharge (blah…)
- You develop a fever (another sign of infection)

Allowing Your Wound to Heal

While I'm sure you'll be anxious to get back to doing things after your operation, do yourself a favour and let your incision(s) heal! It seems obvious but there's a real chance that you'll find yourself faced with some task or household chore that you'd "just like to get done"… Then, boom… it happens. Next is a trip to the Emergency Room and possibly the Operating Room.

It's called *wound dehiscence*. This is a fancy way to say that the stitches or staples have let go and the incision opens up. It's one of the most common problems with surgical wounds and *it could happen to anyone*. The highest risk for this is in the first couple of weeks as your tissues are just beginning to heal back together.

Here are a couple tips to help you prevent this from happening:

PREVENT INFECTION
- Follow the wound care instructions you were given (infection of your wound puts you at greater risk for wound dehiscence)
- Take your antibiotics and other medications as instructed

AVOID STRESS ON THE WOUND

- Ask your surgeon for *specific* instructions about what you can and cannot do (e.g. heavy lifting, exercise and driving), especially during those first couple weeks
- Ask for ways to protect or brace the wound during activity (using a pillow, for example)

Ask your surgeon to be very specific about what activities you can do once you're home, as well as things to avoid. Next, you'll hear a story from a close friend of mine who has endured multiple surgeries. His experience highlights the importance of involving people in your healthcare, especially during the transition home.

In Your Shoes

PHIL'S STORY

We should all be so lucky as to have a friend like Phil. I could easily run down a long list of admirable qualities that would equally describe and embarrass him. I'll spare him this; however, it was a number of these qualities that undoubtedly helped him through a battle that lasted for two years of his life.

It seemed to have all started with a gallbladder attack. Easy fix, right? Take it out. And so it was—a cholecystectomy, as it's called. The surgery went fine; however, recovery at home didn't play out as he was anticipating.

Phil is a pretty tough guy but once home after surgery, his pain began increasing steadily to the point where he wisely went to the Emergency Room at a nearby hospital. This is when the unexpected happened.

The pain wasn't from his gallbladder surgery. It turned out that the swelling from his surgery compressed a tumour that had been silently growing in his colon. This caused a complete blockage of his colon that created the pain he was experiencing.

By the time you read this book, he'll have had his fourth surgery in two years and will have had two rounds of chemotherapy. I'm thrilled (and relieved) to know that he's now doing very well. His optimism and selflessness during this time was remarkable. His generosity now flows to you through the reflections he shared with me during a long drive from Mont-Tremblant, Quebec, to Toronto, Ontario. Let's learn from his experience to make yours better.

Going In

Phil felt like he could have been better prepared for his stay in hospital. Sure, he knew what surgery he was having but didn't have a good idea about what he should or shouldn't bring with him. It turned out that storage was at a minimum during his stay on the Hospital Ward. He realized once he was there that valuables, such as watches, jewelry and electronics, were not very secure.

The lesson here: Plan what to bring. Use your Ready for My Surgery Checklist as a guide and reminder of what you'll need as you prepare to head to the hospital. Leave everything except the essentials at home.

Phil's laptop kept him occupied when he was stuck in bed on the ward. Movies distracted him and helped the time go by. For Patricia, if you recall, it was music. What is it for you? Books, audiobooks, magazines, crossword puzzles, video games, writing—think about what comforts you when you're feeling unwell and how you can bring that comfort with you.

Sure Would Have Been Nice to Know the Plan

Phil really didn't know what the plan was for him during his recovery on the ward. Because of this, he didn't realize what was important to focus on in order to be discharged. It turned out, "that first bowel movement was a big deal"! Who knew? Someone did, just not Phil.

He found himself highly dependent on the nursing staff for medications and knowing what the next step was. Phil's a brilliant, successful business executive—the big picture is his thing! He would have preferred to have understood the overall plan for his care so he could make sure that he was doing everything he could to stay on track.

Is this a reasonable expectation? It is. This situation highlights an opportunity to do things a little better. It takes only a slight shift in an institution's practice and expectations toward patient engagement and empowerment to produce a disproportionately large increase in a patient's participation in their care, as well as their satisfaction with the entire experience. The shift has begun. We'll get there. Being engaged and clear on your expectations will fuel this shift.

Preparing for Home

I could tell that Phil was particularly disappointed about the lack of support and guidance related to his transition from hospital to home. Here's what he wasn't told but wishes he had been:

PREPARING HIS HOME
- Keeping things within easy reach and having pre-prepared home-cooked meals

NUTRITION
- Particularly since he'd just had abdominal surgery, he expected some guidance on the types of foods to eat and those to avoid (other than "don't eat fried foods"—advice that applies to pretty much the entire population…)
- Not until he asked specifically did recommendations regarding vitamins and supplements become available

PREVENTING PROBLEMS
- All he was told about activities to avoid was "Don't lift anything over 10 pounds"… Okay, sure. Why, exactly? The problem with advice like this, according to Phil, is that it doesn't explain the objective or the consequences
- Disappointingly, Phil developed a hernia because some of the internal stitches that closed his wound let go. Could this have been prevented if he'd better understood how to protect it? If he had fully appreciated the consequences of not allowing his incision to heal properly, would he have acted differently? Knowing what he knows now, if he could have acted differently to prevent a hernia and a subsequent painful surgery to fix it, he certainly would have

We're going to have you well prepared for your return home after surgery. Let's keep these things in mind as we do.

Communication Breakdown

You've heard of the situation where someone gets a phone call from their doctor's office saying, "We have your test results back and the doctor wants you to come in right away." That's probably the worst message possible because you're left entirely to speculation and your imagination to fill in the unknowns.

Phil got that call. In typical fashion, he shrugged and went in accepting of whatever he heard. He sure didn't have a warm and fuzzy feeling about it though.

It turned out that his family doctor thought the surgeon had already shared the pathology results with Phil... he didn't. These were the results that would determine whether Phil had cancer or not. Crazy, right?

The tumour was in fact cancerous and it's fair to say that neither Phil nor his doctor were well prepared for the communication of this information. There was a disconnect between hospital and community care, surgeon and family doctor. Not only did he not know the results, but he had no indication of when he'd get the pathology results back (it ended up being a week after he was home). Phil's a particularly resilient, level-headed guy and that's a good thing, because in this case, he didn't have the support of the system.

As you read this, you may be surprised or angry. Maybe annoyed that we're bringing up someone else's problem. There's an expression I'm quite fond of that goes something like this:

"Smart people learn from their mistakes. Wise people learn from other people's mistakes."

Emergency Preparedness

We're not talking about grabbing the canned goods and heading for the basement... though different types of issues (even emergencies) can happen once you're home from surgery. Are you ready? You will be.

Phil developed his hernia at home. Obviously, he was pretty concerned but he wasn't at all clear on what he should do or who to call. Looking back, this is an easy fix—for you, your Ready for My Surgery Checklist will address this.

Your checklist will serve another purpose too. You need to know what constitutes an emergency, where to go and what information is important to provide. This isn't difficult information to get ahead of time. Once you're home though, and you're having some sort of problem, what you need to do in that moment can be a lot less clear.

Before you leave the hospital, the healthcare professionals you are working with can give you this information. Ask them to fill in the checklist for you, if you'd like. With this done, you're now ready to handle much of what could happen.

If you need to go to the Emergency Room (ER), imagine how much easier it would be for the ER team to understand your situation if you hand them your checklist while you describe the issue you're experiencing. Your health history, your surgical history, your allergies and medications… it's all there. It would be easy to underestimate just how valuable this information would be to the ER staff that have just met you and are trying to determine the best course of treatment to help you. You will also avoid forgetting important pieces of information—quite possible in a situation where you may be distracted by the issue at hand.

There were a lot of things that went perfectly well for Phil, most in fact. But we're striving for better here. Having spoken to many patients and reflecting on my years working in the hospital, we're wise to learn from these situations. This is how we get better. This is how we can create a better experience for you and those to follow.

Thanks for sharing, Phil.

Pain After Surgery

Pain after surgery is often the biggest concern of patients, says a research article from a renowned journal called *Anesthesia and Analgesia*.[2]

Is this the case for you? Let's explore this together so you can understand how pain management works and your role in it.

Sharing Your Pain

You will have some discomfort—you just had surgery after all! However, the goal is reduce your discomfort so that it is mild and quite tolerable. You'll need to move around after surgery and great pain control will help you do that.

During your time in the hospital after surgery, you'll be asked to rate your pain. Pain is subjective, meaning that it will simply be your perception of it. Everyone experiences pain differently. Using a standard scale, it is much easier for you to describe the pain you are experiencing in a way that is helpful to the people who are treating you.

The rating is usually based on a scale of 0 to 10 where: 0 = no pain; and 10 = excruciating pain. You may be asked to rate your pain both at rest and when you're moving. Here's a visual rating scale developed by the Wong-Baker FACES

---

[2] Jeffrey L. Apfelbaum et al., "Postoperative Pain Experience: Results from a National Survey Suggest Postoperative Pain Continues to Be Undermanaged." *Anesthesia and Analgesia* (2003), https://www.ncbi.nlm.nih.gov/pubmed/12873949.

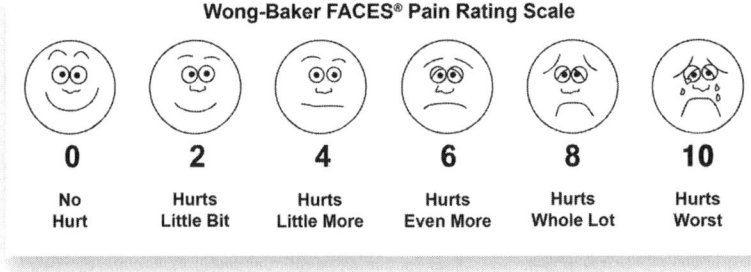

Wong-Baker FACES Foundation (2016). Wong-Baker FACES® Pain Rating Scale. Retrieved February 24, 2017 with permission from https://wongbakerfaces.org

Foundation—this is quite helpful if reading is a challenge for you (e.g. you're not wearing your glasses or if any barriers to communication exist, such as speech or language).

Most hospitals in North America have a team dedicated to managing pain for patients in hospital; this team is usually called the Acute Pain Service. This team works closely with your surgical team to ensure your pain doesn't get in the way of your recovery.

Pain Control & the Importance of Movement

In case you missed it the first time, don't wait until your pain is unbearable to ask for help with managing your pain. No need to be stoic and accept excruciating pain as just part of the deal of having an operation. It isn't.

If you can't do the exercises or activities prescribed to you because of pain, this means that your pain isn't sufficiently controlled. Take knee replacement surgery for example—getting that knee joint moving after surgery is crucial to you getting the best result. If you can't do your exercises properly because of pain, the joint can become stiff and your range of motion is reduced. I've seen this happen to the degree where people have needed to have another spinal anesthetic just so the surgeon could restore the range of motion (using brute force!). Yikes.

If you're having surgery on your chest, back or abdomen, controlling pain is important to help you breathe normally and do deep breathing exercises. After having an anesthetic, most people will have a small amount

> 💡 **INSIDER TIP**
>
> **PAIN MEDICATIONS**
> Pain medications don't work immediately—don't wait for the pain to be too intense before taking a dose. It is more difficult to get severe pain under control than to keep moderate pain under control in the first place. Stick to your prescribed dose but if your pain is not well controlled, be sure to let your nurse or doctor know.
>
> The answer to better pain control isn't always to just increase the dose—the higher the dose, the greater the potential for side effects. It may be that an additional medication is best. There may be other treatments that are even more effective than drugs, such as using ice to reduce and control swelling.
>
> Good control of your pain immediately after an operation (called *acute pain*) is a very important way of preventing you from developing long-term pain (called *chronic pain*). Chronic pain can be debilitating and doing what we can to prevent it is important. Do your part to minimize your discomfort—this includes sticking to the plan for pain control and communicating when it isn't working.

of their lung tissue collapse (this is called *atelectasis*—think of a balloon that has lost its air and needs to be re-inflated). There are a few things that can be done to reduce this during your anesthetic but the odds are that you'll still experience this to some degree.

How will you know?

In general, if your lungs were healthy before surgery (and you didn't have lung surgery specifically) you shouldn't really need oxygen afterward, should you? You didn't need it when you walked into the hospital, right? To make this point clear, almost everyone is given oxygen therapy after an operation and atelectasis is usually to blame. The main way to treat this is to do deep breathing exercises (you'll be taught these in the hospital).

If pain is keeping you from expanding your chest and taking deep breaths, you won't be able to get your lungs back to normal. Not only will you need oxygen therapy longer, you'll also be at higher risk for developing a lung infection... otherwise known as *pneumonia*.

We've also talked about the importance of moving after surgery to prevent blood clots. Blood clots that form in your veins (from not moving enough, or from a clotting disorder) is a condition called *deep vein thrombosis (DVT)*. The risk is highest in the first few weeks after surgery.

These clots usually form in your legs and can break free and travel to another part of the body (called a *thromboembolism*). The lungs are a common place (and a bad place) for these clots to end up—this particular condition is called a *pulmonary embolism*, which blocks one or more arteries in the lungs.

Sounds bad, huh? It sure can be. Keeping the body moving after surgery is important, particularly the lower legs. Be sure to seek medical advice if you have unexplained swelling or pain in your lower leg, even if it's weeks or months after your operation.

Scheduling Your Medications

As far as timing of pain medications is concerned, you can certainly work with your pharmacist, nurse or doctor to figure this out. If you have scheduled activities that cause you pain (therapy, exercises, dressing changes, etc.), it works out very well if you plan to take medications in advance. The tricky part is that different medications take different lengths of time to reach their peak effect. Planned well, your pain control is at its peak when you need it most.

Medication Side Effects

I mentioned side effects during the Insider Tip on pain medications. All prescription pain medications (all medications in general, actually) have the potential to cause side effects. The key for you is to understand what they are. This is why it's on your Ready for My Surgery Checklist. Ask for this information before you leave the hospital. If you don't get these details, ask your pharmacist—they are experts on this topic (obviously... but sometimes we just don't think to ask).

Many pain medications have side effects which can cause people some alarm if they are not aware of them beforehand (especially after you're already home!). So, ask for a little overview of your medications before you are discharged.

Side Effect or Allergic Reaction?

A *side effect* is simply an unwanted effect of a drug on your body. The insert that comes with your medication contains a list of the drug's possible side effects (it's often surprisingly long!). Here are some examples of medication side effects (let your doctor or pharmacist know if you are experiencing a side effect—often it can be reduced or eliminated):

- Constipation
- Muscle aches
- Low energy
- Difficulty sleeping
- Diarrhea
- There is way, way more...

An *allergic reaction* to a drug results from your body putting up a defence against the "foreign substance" floating around in your bloodstream (most drugs move around your body in your blood). Sometimes, it isn't until the second time you take a drug that the reaction occurs—this is because the first time you took it, you "primed" your body to watch out for this invader. When you take it that second time—boom!—your body attacks!

Here are some signs (things you see) and symptoms (things you feel) with a mild allergic reaction:

- Rash
- Itchy skin

A severe allergic reaction is called *anaphylaxis*—this can be life-threatening so take immediate action to seek help if these signs and symptoms occur:

- Hives (different from a rash—with hives, your skin will be swollen/raised, red and may feel bumpy and itchy)
- Swelling in your face and throat
- Difficulty breathing
- Wheezing (a high-pitched whistling sound you can hear when you breathe out)
- Dizziness/light-headedness

Maybe you know of someone who has a severe food allergy and carries an EpiPen® with them? This is the same type of reaction.

If you experience any of the above signs and symptoms of anaphylaxis, consider it an emergency. Depending on the severity of your symptoms, a trip to the Emergency Room or an ambulance is generally your best option.

If you have any type of unexpected or unwanted reaction to a medication, don't keep it to yourself. Here's what to do:

- **If you're in the hospital**, let your nurse or doctor know of your symptoms right away. Getting your medications sorted out before you go home will be of great benefit to you.
- **If you're home**, use your Ready for My Surgery Checklist and call your doctor or pharmacist to let them know your signs and symptoms.

Forms of Pain Control

There are three mains ways that your pain will be looked after using medications. Here's a quick summary of each:

1. *Patient-controlled analgesia (PCA)* is a way for you to give yourself pain medications using special pre-programmed pumps. This can be done either through an IV (i.e. Intravenous Patient-Controlled Analgesia) or through an epidural (i.e. Patient-Controlled Epidural Analgesia).

2. Some surgeries benefit from having a *peripheral nerve block*. This involves one or more injections of a local anesthetic that temporarily block the signals of nerves going to and from certain parts of the body, such as a hand or foot. These can be very helpful in controlling pain, both during and after surgery.

3. Most of the time, you'll be prescribed *oral pain medications* (e.g. pills/tablets) by the time you are ready to go home. Before going home, make sure to have your prescriptions filled—you don't want to be caught without these medications, especially during the time you are transitioning home.

Pain Relief Without Medications

Medications aren't the only way to control pain. A major contributor to pain after surgery is swelling and inflammation. Ask a member of your surgical team if any of the following would be helpful for you:

- Ice and/or heat applied to your wound
- Elevation (e.g. keeping your leg elevated after foot surgery)
- Compression or splinting (e.g. using a pillow for support after abdominal surgery)
- Nutrition (e.g. anti-inflammatory diet)
- Movement (e.g. rehabilitation exercises balanced with appropriate rest)

Your mind has a powerful role to play as well. Mindfulness-based activities are widely used for patients with chronic pain. Consider seeking expert advice regarding techniques to help you reduce stress and take your focus away from the source of pain.

Such techniques include meditation, guided imagery, body awareness and yoga.

5 Questions

Through a collaborative effort, the Institute for Safe Medication Practices (ISMP) Canada has produced a one-page document that is valuable for every person taking medications (whether you're in Canada or not!). This doesn't just apply when you're having surgery, these questions are important anytime you're taking medications. Medication safety and error prevention work best when you (*the one taking the drugs*) are armed with the essential information. With permission, the next page features this resource, called "5 Questions to Ask About Your Medications."

Tests After Surgery

Here are some of the common tests you may have while in hospital:

- Blood work
- X-ray
- CT scan
- MRI
- Ultrasound

You should always be informed as to why a test is being performed. If it is unclear, it is your right to ask questions—in fact, I'd say it's your responsibility.

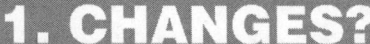

5 Questions to Ask About Your Medications Working Group. 5 Questions to Ask About Your Medications. Toronto, ON: Institute for Safe Medication Practices Canada; 2016. Produced in collaboration with Canadian Patient Safety Institute (CPSI), Patients for Patient Safety Canada (PFPSC), Institute for Safe Medication Practices Canada (ISMP Canada), Canadian Society of Hospital Pharmacists (CSHP), Canadian Pharmacists Association (CPhA). Available at https://www.ismp-canada.org/medrec/5questions.htm. Accessed January 7, 2017.

Hospital Visitors

There will be certain times during the day when you can visit with family and friends—this is a great way to help the time go by a little quicker, especially if you are in bed much of the time. It's helpful for your loved ones to know the policy on visitors beforehand so that they can best time their visits.

A simple rule for visitors: Treat a hospital visit as you would a visit to someone's home—be courteous, respectful and considerate.

Infection Prevention & Control

Infections at the site of surgery are the most common type of infection people get after an operation. Are these infections a big deal?

Unfortunately, yes.

For example, you are five times more likely to end up back in the hospital if you get this type of infection. Not good.

Most of the responsibility in preventing these infections rests with your Surgical and Anesthesia Care Teams. They are charged to make sure:

1. Your site of surgery is **properly cleaned and prepared**
5. You are **kept warm** (before, during and after surgery)
6. Your **blood sugar is controlled** (for diabetics)
7. **Appropriate antibiotics** are given and stopped at appropriate times

Once you are able to move about and start caring for yourself, your work begins in helping to prevent yourself from acquiring an infection, as well as preventing the spread of germs to others. Here's how:

- Wash your hands
- Ask your care providers if they have washed their hands
- Ask your visitors to wash their hands
- If you have diabetes, keep your blood sugar (glucose) under control
- If you smoke, quitting before surgery reduces your risk of infection

Don't underestimate the importance of hand-washing—antibiotic-resistant germs are dangerous and this is one of the best and easiest ways for you to avoid infection.

Check out the infographic on the next page from the Association for Professionals in Infection Control and Epidemiology; it gives give you some key tips on preventing infection in hospital.

Recovery in the Intensive Care Unit (ICU)

Does your surgery or pre-existing state of health warrant a higher level of care and treatment than a Hospital Ward is designed to provide?

Enter the ICU.

An Intensive Care Unit is a specialty department within a hospital designed to care for patients who require continuous monitoring and active treatment of conditions that pose an immediate threat to their health. It's a serious place, no doubt.

Why might *you* end up here after surgery?

Here are some situations that fit the bill:

COMPLEX SURGERY

Complex can mean different things in surgery:

- Sometimes surgery can be very long (I've witnessed some that started one day at 8:00 a.m. and ended the next day!)

- Some surgeries are very invasive and can make a significant change to the functioning of the body (e.g. lung or liver transplantation)

- Some surgeries are complex and delicate and require specialized monitoring afterward (e.g. neurosurgery)

EMERGENCY SURGERY

This category includes any type of injury or disease state causing an immediate threat to someone's life that requires immediate surgery

- Examples include trauma caused by motor vehicle accidents or rupture of an aneurysm (an enlarged, weakened artery—usually in the head or abdomen)

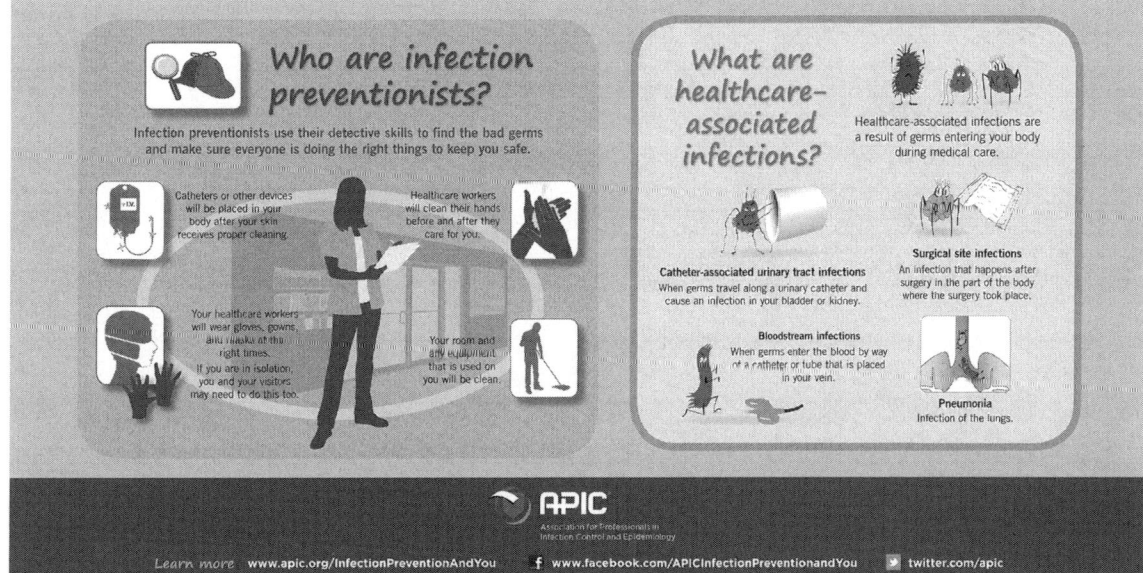

Association for Professionals in Infection Control and Epidemiology (2017). Infection Control and You. Retrieved February 24, 2017 with permission from http://apic.org

COMPLICATIONS WITH SURGERY (more on this shortly)

OTHER
- Life threatening conditions, such as traumatic injuries or medical crises
- Disease states or infections that have worsened to the point where constant medical care and intervention is required

Large university teaching hospitals will have multiple specialty ICUs. Here are some examples:

- **Cardiovascular ICU**—(*cardio = heart; vascular = blood vessels*) for patients recovering from cardiac (heart) surgery

- **Neurosurgical ICU**—(*neuro = nervous system, including the brain and spinal cord*) for patients recovering from surgeries on the brain and spinal cord

- **Medical-Surgical ICU**—for patients with life-threatening medical conditions (such as severe infections or breathing problems) as well as post-surgery patients (such as surgery on the lung, liver, major blood vessels and transplants)

- **Coronary ICU**—(*coronary = arteries and veins of the heart*) for patients with heart conditions, such as heart failure and heart attacks

- **Trauma ICU**—for patients who have been in injured in accidents (anything from car accidents to violent crimes)

Complications

Every single professional involved in your care has the common goal of ensuring your surgery goes smoothly and as planned. As in every other part of life though, sometimes we're thrown curveballs. A curveball during surgery may result in admission to ICU to manage the unplanned troublesome situation. A common fear relates to being the one to whom something unplanned occurs—let's explore that idea a little.

As you would expect, this topic is very closely studied. The rate of surgical complications is generally low and each type of procedure and hospital has its own statistics. To come to a place of acceptance with this, simply ask yourself:

What aspects of my care can I control?

Answer this question and then do your part. Expect to be a partner in your care and work together with your healthcare team. This will ensure you know what actions you need to take. Leave the rest to the professionals and be at peace with this. On a team, every person has a role and relies on their teammates to do their part. Accept what you cannot control—once you do, focus on being grateful that you have access to the care you need. When you step on a plane, you know there is a small chance that something won't go as planned but you trust in the people and the process.

Same idea.

So, what can I control? If you've gotten this far into the book, you already know. And you're already *taking* control. As a recap, you are:

- Optimizing your health before surgery

- Understanding and following the instructions given to you and are asking questions if something doesn't make sense

- Making sure you take your medications as instructed

- Making sure you don't take the medications you are told not to take

- Educating yourself and preparing to seek clarification (questioning things that don't sound right), and expecting to be an active participant in your cares

How Your Care Is Different in the ICU
ONE-TO-ONE NURSING CARE
- ICU nurses receive specialty training in order to manage the complicated care that they must provide

- Highly-focused medical specialists actively diagnose, monitor and treat life-threatening conditions

  - The sickest of patients require specialists that can manage multiple medical challenges at the same time

  - Life-threatening crises are not uncommon in the ICU—the knowledge and skills required to manage these takes years of preparation

BREATHING SUPPORT IS COMMON
- For patients who can no longer breathe adequately on their own, it is possible to artificially support breathing—this is called *mechanical ventilation*

- "Breathing machines" called *mechanical ventilators* (sometimes misnamed "respirators") are used to support some or all of a person's breathing—these are the devices commonly referred to as *life support*

- This type of therapy requires continuous monitoring, in-depth knowledge of how the lungs and related organs work, the nature of the condition(s) causing the breathing problem and the interaction with all other treatments

- In North America, Respiratory Therapists take on this challenge. In other parts of the world, doctors and ICU nurses primarily manage this therapy

TEAM APPROACH
- Although teamwork is an integral part of every hospital department, the complicated, ever-changing nature of patient care in the ICU requires all professionals to work diligently together toward common goals for the patient

- This happens through continuous evaluation of each patient and daily team discussions—this is critical to achieving the best outcome

- The patient and family are part of this team—discussions should happen with you, not just in front of you. The next chapter will help you contribute to the growth of your healthcare system when you find this not to be true.

Lives are saved in the ICU, that's for certain. It's an intense, demanding and rewarding place.

Recovery at Home

I'm outta here!
Walk, don't run...

Excited, right? Maybe that's not the right word. Relieved? Sure, but perhaps a little hesitant too?

You *are* leaving all the healthcare professionals behind, along with their answers to your questions and the timely directions that were keeping you on the right path to a good recovery.

To help you feel better prepared to go home, all we have to do is get your questions answered and your plan laid out for you before you leave the hospital. No sweat. Here's how we'll do it:

1. Pull out your Ready for My Surgery Checklist

2. Ask your healthcare team to help you complete the "My Appointments" and "My Recovery" sections. Here's some of what we'll write down:

    - Follow-up appointments
    - Average time to a full recovery
    - How to care for your incision(s)/wound(s)
    - Pain medications and side effects
    - Special equipment for home (e.g. bandages, crutches, bathroom accessories, etc.)
    - Exercises and therapy to help with your recovery
    - Activities to avoid and why
    - Issues you may experience at home (e.g. swelling, bruising, etc.)
    - Follow-up tests and test results
    - Return to work and any work-related restrictions
    - Who to call if you have concerns once you're home
    - When to seek urgent care (i.e. go to the Emergency Room)

And many more things that you'll most certainly forget... It really is a lot to think about. Who can remember all this?

That's why a checklist makes it so much easier. Just ask your healthcare team to help you fill in the blanks. This is a great task to delegate to a family member! It's important that you know this stuff but you shouldn't need to memorize it.

Fortunately, most hospitals have a clear process for discharging you. Sometimes though, a lot of instructions are given to you verbally (not great if you've just had sedation or anesthesia—remember its effect on your memory?). You could also end up with a pile of different forms and booklets. One master checklist will help you organize your thoughts and ask the important questions.

The main thing is that you have all the vital information you need—*at home*. It's not so easy to get quick answers to questions from healthcare professionals once you've left the hospital. So, let's get them while you can.

Catching a Ride

In your planning, you've wisely arranged for someone to take you home from the hospital. Depending on your operation and the type of anesthetic you've had, you may need someone to stay with you overnight for a period of time. Your healthcare team will let you know how long. This is in the checklist too.

Who Will Support You Once You Get Home?

Ideally, there will be strong communication between the hospital staff planning your discharge and the people and resources available to you in your community. Your checklist has a section related to this—ask for the contact information of your community resources to be added. This is a topic worth talking about with your family doctor or surgeon before the surgery.

Here are some of the resources you may have available to you at home:

- Community care coordinators (these professionals coordinate your home care services during and after your transition home from the hospital)
- Community care, or "home care" (such as physiotherapy, occupational therapy, nursing, respiratory therapy, etc.)
- Family doctor (some family doctors still do home visits! That's awesome)
- Pharmacist (just a phone call away)
- Surgeon's office (follow-up visits)
- Friends and family (can be some of the best help around)

Your expectations regarding collaboration, professionalism, infection control and quality of care should be the same regardless of where you interact with your healthcare system and its professionals. Your communication and feedback regarding your home care services are as important as when you are in hospital—don't hesitate to offer both positive and constructive feedback about your home care experience.

The Comforts (and Discomforts) of Home

Ah, back home. It can be such a relief to step back into a familiar environment to rest and recover. Rest and *recover*. It's understanding that recovery piece that's the key to optimizing the ultimate outcome of your surgery from here on in.

Rehabilitation is probably a better word than recovery—it's really about restoring yourself to good health, the best that is possible for your situation. You understand the importance of being active in your recovery—we've talked about exercise and movement a little already. Once you arrive home, you'll need to motivate yourself to keep up the activities prescribed to you. This isn't always easy.

Your Why

Some surgeries take more effort to recover from than others. Sometimes, it's a long and challenging process. How can you stay motivated? The answer is different for everyone—this is because each of us is motivated by something different. This is our *why*.

Maybe it's being available for your kids, your grandkids or your spouse/partner. Perhaps getting back to your job or your business is your driver. Many people give of their time to charities and other causes which offers them a great source of joy and motivation. Whatever it is for you, name it.

This is your *why*.

Remind yourself of your why whenever you need some extra motivation. As with any journey, there can be hard parts. Knowing your why is one of the best ways to help you push through and finish strong.

Here are some of the things that can become hard:

- Exercise and therapy
- Pain control
- Eating well
- Changes in appearance
- Smoking, alcohol and other substances
- Getting back to daily work and life
- Financial impact of healthcare and time away from work
- Personal relationships (e.g. your *guilt* of feeling like a burden; their *resentment* of having to do so much more to care for you)
- Your psychology (Are you *allowing* yourself to dwell on the negatives and the things you don't have? Or, are you *focused* on your why and the opportunity this situation presents?)

Just being aware of these things can help you identify when they're slowing you down.

Stronger, Faster, Healthier

We talked about this earlier—you know, the getting healthy spiel. It's up to you, of course, but the benefits are undeniable; you will never regret taking the opportunity to improve your health. The time is now and you've never had more resources to help you along the way.

There are three main areas that you may like to address:

1. Fitness & Exercise
8. Healthy Eating & Nutrition
9. Quitting Smoking (once and for all)

Creating new routines and habits are challenging. Motivation can quickly wane... This is why I've addressed each of these topics in three separate podcast episodes. I've interviewed experts related to each topic—each is full of practical advice to support your efforts and help you achieve your goals. Visit www.readyformysurgery.com to see these and many other episodes to help you prepare, engage and recover.

Fitness & Exercise

From elite athletes returning to their sport, to the elderly readying themselves to again play with their grandchildren, fitness and exercise are important after surgery but will mean different things for different people. During the *Ready for My Surgery* podcast, I'll introduce you to experts in the field of exercise and fitness to share their strategies of rehabilitation and strength-building. You can use this knowledge to work with your healthcare professionals to craft an exercise program fit for you.

Healthy Eating & Nutrition

This topic also needs to meet your individual needs. How important is it? Just flip back to the "Eating Well" section earlier in this chapter for a refresher. We're not satisfied with good nutrition just in and around the time of your surgery; this is an opportunity to make some new habits around food.

I'd love for you to explore this topic with me as I speak with nutrition experts on the *Ready for My Surgery* podcast. Appendix D walks you through everything offered for you at www.readyformysurgery.com.

Quitting Smoking

We tackled the topic of smoking in Chapter 1—Scheduled for Surgery. I've dedicated a podcast episode to support anyone interested in learning more, whether you're ready to quit or just curious about the options available to you should you want to quit down the road. It turns out, the road of longevity may become longer for those who quit...

Here's to a Great Recovery!

I hope your journey through recovery is smooth and you achieve the outcome you were expecting. If you've gotten this far in the book before your operation, you may benefit from re-reading this section again after your surgery. I hope you find the information here to be helpful and encouraging.

Carry on to the last chapter to find out how you can share your feedback and experiences to help:

1. Ready for My Surgery continue to grow and improve.
10. Your healthcare institution and its staff to grow and improve.
11. Patients who follow you to benefit from improvements you've helped to shape.

5

GIVING FEEDBACK & GIVING BACK

PURPOSE OF THIS CHAPTER
To encourage you to consider participating in the growth and evolution of your healthcare system by sharing your experience, insight and ideas.

KEY THINGS WE'LL COVER
- The unique value you have the potential to share
- The impact of feedback
- Getting your message across
- Giving back to get better – the power of giving

I'VE HAD THE privilege of spending time in numerous Operating Rooms across Canada over the years. I've provided anesthesia care to patients having surgery and I've been an educator of new advanced anesthesia technologies to anesthesiologists and their teams. These turned out to be wonderful opportunities to observe patients and their care as they experienced surgery.

It's one thing to observe. It's another to experience.

This is what makes your perspective as a patient so valuable. Years of professional training cannot stand in for *actually being a patient—actually having surgery*.

I spent the first few days of my first year of high school in a bed on my Community Hospital ward. The Sunday before my first day of grade nine I started having terrible pain in my abdomen. A few hours later I had moved through the local Emergency Room, enjoyed my first general anesthetic and left the OR short one appendix. I had an appendectomy, as it's called.

I do have a couple vivid memories of that day. It all went pretty well for me, as far as I can recall. Looking back, my experience *was* unique; not that there aren't many other people who have had their appendix removed, even in an emergency such as mine. My interactions with hospital staff; my experience waiting in the ER; my experience as a 14-year-old during the times I was alone on the Hospital Ward; my experience dealing with the discomfort (on multiple levels) of moving slowly around the halls of my new high school, one week late for the party—all these experiences belong to me. And from them, lessons could be learned. I was not asked for my feedback, though. But that was then, this is now.

What Lessons Could Be Learned from Your *Experiences?*

Imagine the type of transformation that would be possible if your experience of surgery, ideas for change and reinforcement of what worked was *combined* with the thousands of other patients who move through the system every day. This is where the power is—giving every person a voice and channelling key messages to a system that needs your direction.

How can this be done? This is a larger goal of Ready for My Surgery—I want to capture the voices from every patient I can. When the right questions are asked to enough people, themes begin to emerge. These themes become pointers—pointers to leaders within healthcare that can help to steer their leadership toward the types of practices and policies that improve care.

What is my ask of you? A survey. That's it.

If you're already receiving emails from me, you'll get an email with a link to an online survey. If not, visit www.readyformysurgery.com and subscribe. You give your honest feedback and thoughtful suggestions and I'll work to find and share the themes and ideas that emerge.

I hope you take a few minutes to share. It could create a better experience—even a better outcome—for others in the future (maybe even someone close to you).

Feedback for Your Hospital

Some feedback you'll have will be very specific to either your hospital or one of its staff. When this is the case, a survey aiming to make large system changes isn't really the right avenue.

Every hospital has a department that will handle specific feedback from their patients and families, good and bad. This department may be called Patient and Family Relations, for example. Online feedback forms are available on some hospital websites too.

If you feel that a hospital or a particular individual would do well to receive specific feedback regarding their performance, head to the hospital website to find the right path to take. As an alternative, simply call the main hospital telephone number and ask to be connected to patient relations.

Saying Thanks

From the perspective of a healthcare professional, to receive a compliment from a patient is tremendously rewarding. If you feel that someone you worked with during your journey through surgery deserves acknowledgement, go out of your way to make it known. Written letters and emails are the best ways to have your message shared with an individual and their superiors.

The benefits of this go beyond the warm feelings. By highlighting behaviours or activities that benefitted you, you are reinforcing those actions—making it much more likely that they will be repeated.

Elaborate—give the details. Tell your story. You'd be surprised by the impact it could have.

Constructive Criticism

You may be disappointed in some aspect(s) of your care. I hope this isn't the case, but it does happen.

There's a reason I didn't title this section "Complaints"—here's why: Complaining is essentially sharing an issue with someone who can't do anything about it. From this point of view, complaining serves no useful purpose; it only prolongs your suffering from whatever happened to you.

Since you can't change something that has already happened and complaining doesn't get you anywhere, how can you best handle an experience that wasn't acceptable? Constructive criticism.

There's research on this topic that highlights the best ways to give constructive feedback to healthcare institutions to improve the likelihood that change will happen. And that's the goal, isn't it? For change to be made so that an unwanted error/behaviour/process doesn't happen again. It's a really good reason to follow through on giving constructive criticism. It may also lift the burden of that experience from your shoulders so that you can more easily move on from it.

There are a number of evidence-based suggestions regarding giving feedback to promote general healthcare practice improvement—we can take a few of these recommendations to improve the feedback that we give:[1]

- Give feedback as soon as possible
- Be specific about the actions that could be improved
- Focus on changes that would be under the recipient's control
- Provide feedback in a way that reduces the likelihood of a defensive reaction

---

1 Jamie C. Brehaut et al. "Practice Feedback Interventions: 15 Suggestions for Optimizing Effectiveness." *Annals of Internal Medicine* (2016), https://www.ncbi.nlm.nih.gov/pubmed/26903136.

Valuable Types of Feedback

There's no wrong answer—no *wrong* feedback (though, how you frame it will influence how it is received).

If you're wondering about what types of feedback would be most helpful, here are a few examples to get the wheels turning:

Communication (in every area)
- *Positive feedback:* "I felt like my surgeon went out of their way to sit with me on the morning of surgery and not only reviewed the plan for surgery but made sure I expressed any questions or concerns I had. I felt like she was sincerely interested in my needs and perspectives as a person, not just her next patient."

- *Constructive criticism:* "After my surgery, I was waiting to be discharged but it took longer than I expected. I didn't know the reason for the delay and what I could do about it. I felt disconnected and disappointed by this."

Processes (did the system work smoothly or did it break somewhere along the way?)
- *Positive feedback:* "Before going home I was clearly told what to do, what to watch out for, what to do if I needed help and was given all the information I needed regarding my follow-up appointments. It was very reassuring to see how well my care was transitioned from hospital to home."

- *Constructive criticism:* "I felt very dependent on the staff in the hospital for information and direction. I was often unsure of what my next step would be. I expected that I would have been moved efficiently from the xxxxxx (e.g. Emergency Room) to the xxxxxx (e.g. Operating Room) but the delay was greater than seemed reasonable."

Professionalism (by all staff)

- *Positive feedback:* "My xxxxxx (healthcare professional) was very thorough in going through all of the therapy I needed to do at home and thoughtfully answered all of my questions. I felt reassured by their knowledge and compassion for my situation."

- *Constructive criticism:* "I found that a number of conversations about my care happened in front of me but not with me when I was in xxxxxx department (e.g. ward, OR, etc.). That made me feel xxxxxx (e.g. frustrated, angry, disappointed)."

Environment (privacy, noise, security, cleanliness)
- *Positive feedback:* "The environment on the ward was quiet, clean and very conducive to recovering from my operation. I appreciated the respect shown for my privacy and need for rest."

- *Constructive criticism:* "I felt like my personal information was being discussed openly and within earshot of other patients while I was in the Pre-Operative Area. I would recommend that more sensitivity to this be taken in the future."

Surgery and Anesthesia (your experience)
- *Positive feedback:* "The staff that walked me into the Operating Room were wonderful. Each person greeted me warmly and made me feel welcome and important. I went off to sleep much more at ease as a result."

- *Constructive criticism:* "The Operating Room was noisy when I walked in and no one seemed to notice when I came in. Although I had prepared myself well for the operation, I was disappointed by the lack of communication and support I received."

Share your experience and ideas for change. Make it better for the next person.

Giving Back

Perhaps you will be given something valuable during your interaction with your healthcare system. I hope so. In the moment, it can be difficult to appreciate and feel grateful for the care you received. The time around your surgery can be stressful; it's easy to miss the dedicated efforts of the hospital staff working to provide you with the best experience they could.

You're through it now. And looking back is a good thing. Do you see value in the work being done by your hospital?

I've included a section about giving back because I've seen firsthand the impact it has. A great deal is accomplished as a result of contributions offered by the community a hospital serves. Often, the types of projects undertaken by healthcare institutions wouldn't be possible without the generosity of people like you.

It's not just about money. The majority of people don't have the resources to fund a new wing for their hospital. Smaller contributions to hospital lotteries and other fundraisers are a good way to give a few dollars if you can. It all adds up to make a real difference. Don't get me wrong, if you are in a position fortunate enough to help build a hospital wing—and you give for the right reasons—you'll undoubtedly feel wonderful about your remarkable contribution!

Another meaningful and rewarding way to support your hospital is to volunteer your time.

Would You Consider Giving a Little Bit of Your Time?
Maybe you give of your time already—coaching your kid's soccer team or helping to run a local charity fundraiser. Hospitals need volunteers too. If your surgery was performed in your local hospital, you'll have a great perspective on the value it provides. Hospitals are increasingly seeking patients and family members to participate in the planning of patient services and programs, commonly through Patient and Family Advisory Councils. These committees may go by different names but exist to integrate the experience and perspective of patients and their families into discussions and planning related to patient care, research and ways to improve the overall patient experience.

Are you good at organizing people or managing projects? Maybe there's a place for you to help them reach their next fundraising goal.

Do you enjoy meeting new people? Perhaps you can see yourself helping patients find their way at the hospital Information Desk.

Are you an experienced executive or successful entrepreneur? The hospital Board of Directors may be in need of someone just like you.

Is this something you would enjoy? If you find the hospital environment interesting and think you would enjoy spending time contributing to the future success of your local hospital, you should check out the opportunities that await you. A little time on the phone or on your hospital's website will get you started. Good luck and have fun!

Final Thoughts

We've come a long way. You now have the power to influence the outcome of your surgery. You have the knowledge to walk confidently into the hospital feeling prepared and in control.

Don't underestimate just how important this could be.

There is a real possibility that you may need to advocate for yourself if something isn't going as expected. You may need to correct an error in understanding by a healthcare professional. Or, you may not. Everything may—and probably will—go just as planned. In this case, what you know will allow you to feel much more relaxed as the flurry of activities occur.

Peace of mind and a sense of control—I hope this book has imparted some of this to you.

I've seen thousands of patients walk into an Operating Room for surgery. Most were not nearly as prepared as you are now. My goal with Ready for My Surgery is to support a shift so that highly prepared and engaged patients become the norm. I believe this will be an expectation of patients in the future.

Thank you sincerely for spending this time with me. I wish you all the best for a successful surgery and a strong recovery. If you would like, it would be an honour for me to hear how this book has served you. Please feel free to drop me an email at patrick.nellis@readyformysurgery.com.

> *"There is one consolation in being sick; and that is the possibility that you may recover to a better state than you were ever in before."*
> HENRY DAVID THOREAU

ACKNOWLEDGEMENTS

THIS PROJECT HAS been made so much richer and valuable through the thoughtful review, input and guidance of the many people who believed in the value of this book and the importance of empowering patients and families during their journey through surgery.

I have tremendous gratitude for the generous contributions of the following people for helping me build this book into a resource I'm proud to share with patients, their families and caregivers, and healthcare professionals alike:

- Scot Jones
- Dana Oakes
- Dr. Claude LaFlamme
- Dr. Paul Tumber
- Dr. Ahtsham Niazi
- Dr. Lucie Filteau
- Dr. Kevin Lumb
- Bonnie McLeod
- Rupinder Khotar
- Phil Speed
- Patricia Melykuty
- Elizabeth & Jeff Nellis (aka Mom & Dad)
- Nick Kolozetti
- Paul Smith
- Canadian Patient Safety Institute
  - Carla Williams, Ioana Popescu, Tricia Swartz, Gina Peck, Chris Power

- Patients for Patient Safety Canada
  - Laurie Jenkins, Kim Neudorf, Donna Harold, Donna Penner
- Canadian Society of Respiratory Therapists
  - Dr. Andrew West, Carolyn McCoy
- Respiratory Therapy Society of Ontario
  - Dilshad Moosa, Shawna MacDonald, Rob Bryan
- Page Two
  - Trena White, Gabrielle Narsted, Peter Cocking, Jesse Finkelstein
- Organizations that shared resources found throughout the book
  - Choosing Wisely Canada
  - Canadian Patient Safety Institute
  - Canadian Anesthesiologists' Society
  - Institute for Safe Medication Practices Canada
  - Wong-Baker FACES Foundation
  - Association for Professionals in Infection Control and Epidemiology

APPENDIX A
READY FOR MY SURGERY CHECKLIST

READY FOR MY SURGERY CHECKLIST

My Hospital

☐
Hospital/Clinic Name: _____
Address: _____
Main Phone Number: _____
Surgical Admission Phone Number: _____
Website: www. _____ ☐ Did you browse the website? **Y / N**
Hospital Parking Rate: _____
Alternate Parking Options: _____

☐	Hospital/Clinic Type	☐ University Teaching Hospital ☐ Community Hospital ☐ Ambulatory Surgery Centre
☐	Travel Planning	Planned Route: Alternate Route:

My Surgery

☐	Surgery Description	Name of your surgery: _____ Side of surgery (right/left): _____ Comments: _____
☐	Day of Surgery	Date: _____ Person Taking Me? _____ Time: _____ Their Phone #: _____ Check-in Location: _____ Pick-up Time/Date: _____
☐	What is your single biggest concern or challenge related to your surgery?	Concern/Challenge: Who can help?
☐	Surgical Safety Checklist	Will the Surgical Safety Checklist be used during my surgery? **Y / N** If no, can I request that it be used? **Y / N**
☐	Risks	Is there a chance that I may need a blood transfusion? **Y / N** What are the risks associated with my surgery? What is the complication rate associated with my surgery?

My Surgeon

☐ Surgeon's Name: _____
Office Address: _____
Office Phone Number: _____
Surgeon's Website/Email: _____

☐ Information and special instructions from my surgeon:
_____
_____
_____

My Appointments

☐	Pre-Admission Clinic	Date: _____ Time: _____	Appt. Location: _____ Person Helping Me: _____
☐	Medical Test #1: _____	Date: _____ Time: _____	Appt. Location: _____ Person Helping Me: _____
☐	Medical Test #2: _____	Date: _____ Time: _____	Appt. Location: _____ Person Helping Me: _____
☐	Surgeon Follow-up	Date: _____ Time: _____	Appt. Location: _____ Person Helping Me: _____
☐	Family Doctor Follow-up	Date: _____ Time: _____	Appt. Location: _____ Person Helping Me: _____

My Health

☐	Height & Weight	Your height: _____ (cm/inches) Your weight: _____ (kg/lbs)
☐	Medical Conditions	List your medical conditions: _____ _____ _____ Any hospital admissions for these conditions? If so, what happened? When? _____
☐	Previous Surgeries	List any previous surgeries and anesthetics: _____ Have you ever had problems with anesthesia? If so, what happened? When? _____ Has anyone in your family ever had problems with anesthesia? If so, what happened? When? _____
☐	Allergies & Sensitivities	1. Allergies & Sensitivities: 2. List your medication and environmental allergies and sensitivities: _____ 3. Describe the reaction you have: _____

☐	Medication List (include over-the-counter drugs, vitamins & herbal remedies)	List Your Medications (drug/dose/frequency): _____ _____ _____ _____ _____ _____ Has the dose of any medications changed recently? **Y / N** If yes, list changes: _____
☐	Exercise Tolerance	How many fights of stairs can you climb without stopping? ____ flights
☐	Smoking	Do you smoke: **Y / N** If yes, how many years: ____ Packs/day: ____
☐	Smoking Cessation	1. Have you been told to stop smoking prior to your surgery? **Y / N** 2. If yes, how many weeks before? ____ weeks 3. What support and tools will you use to help you quit? _____ _____ 4. Have you sought help to quit smoking for good? **Y / N** 5. If yes, what is your plan: _____ _____ 6. If no, list the internal objections you have to quitting and reasons why you should not take this excellent opportunity to improve your health: _____ _____
☐	Alcohol	Do you drink alcohol: **Y / N** If yes, how many drinks per day: ____

Day of Surgery

☐	Name and phone number of your pharmacy	Name:	Phone:
☐	Name and phone number of your family doctor	Name:	Phone:
☐	Name and phone number of an emergency contact	Name:	Phone:
☐	Insurance Information	Provider & Policy #:	Private / Semi-Private (circle one)
☐	Your Health Card		
☐	Your Hospital Card		
☐	Your medications (in their original packaging)		
☐	Letter from your family doctor & any medical test reports (x-ray, CT scan, MRI, ultrasound, etc.)		

	Other Things to Bring
☐	Clothes (housecoat, comfortable socks, shoes and slippers—for overnight stays)
☐	Toiletries (toothpaste, toothbrush, hair brush, soap, shampoo, scent-free moisturizers, etc.)
☐	Special items (eyeglasses/case, hearing aids/case, walker, cane, CPAP device, etc.)
☐	Entertainment (smartphone & headphones, tablet/laptop, books, magazines, etc.)
☐	Small amount of cash (for food, drinks, TV rental in room, etc.)
☐	Acceptance and gratitude ☺

	My Recovery	
☐	Where will I recover immediately after surgery? ☐ Home ☐ Hospital Ward ☐ Intensive Care Unit	
☐	How long should a full recovery take? ___ weeks. Expected back-to-work date: _____	
☐	Wound Care/ Infection Control	How should I care for my wound(s)? What are signs of infection or problems with the wound(s)?
☐	Medication Side Effects	What new medications have I been prescribed? What medication side effects might I experience? How should I handle these?
☐	Help at Home	Does someone need to stay with me overnight? Y / N How long? ___ nights What special services or equipment do I need? How will communication occur between the hospital and my community care resources?
☐	Exercise, Therapy & Activity Restrictions	What exercises and therapies should I continue at home? What activities/movements should I avoid? Why? When can I resume normal activities? (e.g. lifting, driving, etc.)
☐	Nutrition	What foods, vitamins and supplements will best help me recover?
☐	Challenges & Complications	What complications could arise once I'm home? How can I manage these? When should I go to the Emergency Room? Call an ambulance? What other challenges might I face during my recovery?

Notes

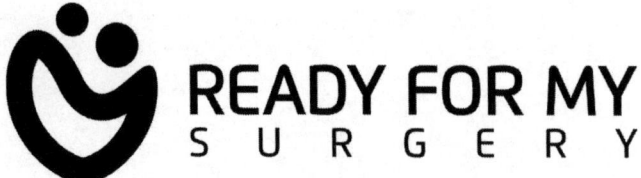

www.readyformysurgery.com

APPENDIX B
MEDICAL TESTS

HERE IS A BRIEF description of some of the common diagnostic tests that may be required of you. Consider this section as a reference. Read through it if you're interested, otherwise, feel free to skip tests that don't apply to your situation (there isn't a quiz at the end ☺).

X-ray

This test uses radiation to generate an image of the body's internal structures.

How It Works

X-ray beams are sent through a part of the body (the image to the right is a chest x-ray) and are absorbed based on the density of that tissue. Bone shows up as white (most absorption), lungs are black (least absorption—because they are filled with air) and other tissues end up being different shades of grey. Fifty, more or less...

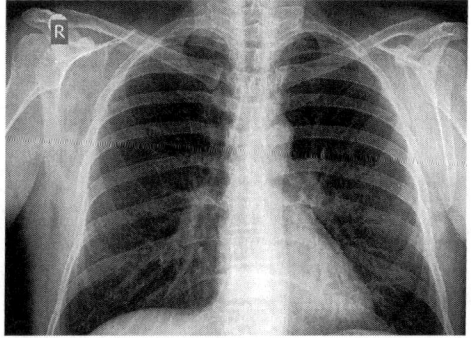

Radiation is dangerous. However, the amount used in a single x-ray is minimal, well below amounts known to cause harm. Having lots of x-rays over time can have more of a cumulative effect and may increase risk of harm.

Sometimes, it is necessary to use a contrast material to better visualize certain body structures in an x-ray. Contrast agents are typically swallowed or injected through an IV prior to the x-ray. They prevent x-ray beams from passing through the selected part of the body and help to better define that body structure. There are some possible side effects from contrast that range from itching, to a metallic taste in your mouth, to a drop in blood pressure. These risks will be discussed with you prior to the test so that you may give informed consent.

Computerized Tomography (CT) Scan

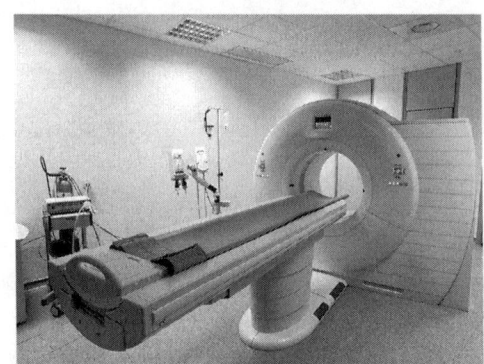

How It Works
This test uses computer processing to combine views from a series of x-rays. The result is a number of cross-sectional images of your internal structures.

Picture this...
Imagine cutting an apple into very thin slices from top to bottom. Each slice will show how the inside of the apple changes throughout its length. Now imagine being able to see each slice without having to cut the apple—that is the essence of the CT scan.

The dose of radiation is much higher than an x-ray. Discussing the risk of this test with your doctor or the staff in the radiology department is important to allow you to give informed consent.

Magnetic Resonance Imaging (MRI)

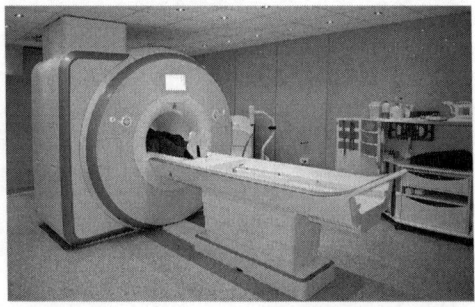

How It Works
An MRI doesn't use radiation. This test uses a powerful magnet to generate images of your body. The MRI machine is built like a tunnel. You'll lay on the

bed as it's moved into the tunnel containing the magnet where images are then captured. This test can take anywhere from ten minutes to more than two hours, depending on the reason for the test.

TEST TIPS

The tough part about this test is that you'll need to keep quite still while the images are being captured. It's also a small space. If you have difficulty managing in tight spaces (e.g. claustrophobia), you'll want to mention this prior to the test. Oh, and it's pretty loud... You'll be given ear protection to wear during the test.

Due to the strong magnetic force, special screening is done for everyone entering the MRI room. Any metal brought into the room can be dangerous as it can fly into the magnet! So, you'll be asked a series of questions before you can enter.

Some common questions include:

- Are you carrying anything with metal?
  - Examples: coins, pens, jewellery, eyeglasses, hair accessories, etc.
- Do you have any metal in your body?
  - Examples: pins, shrapnel, pacemaker, screw implants, piercings, hearing aids, artificial heart valves, aneurysm clips, artificial joints, etc.

Prior to arriving for this test, leave loose metal items at home. If you have any doubts about materials used for past surgeries, clarify this with your doctor ahead of time to prevent delays in having your MRI test.

Ultrasound

There are lots of applications for ultrasound in healthcare. The most familiar are the routine ultrasounds expectant mothers enjoy that monitor the health of their baby. Ultrasound can also be used to image the heart, nerves, blood vessels and organs within the abdomen.

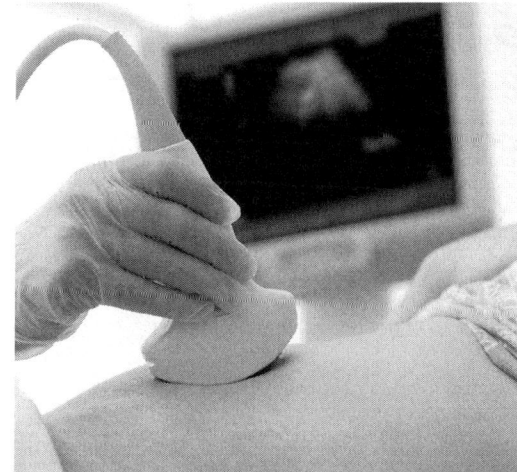

How It Works
This is another test that does not use radiation. Instead, it uses high frequency sound waves to create images of structures inside your body. A small amount of a special ultrasound gel is applied to the skin and the ultrasound probe. The probe is then pressed against the skin where it sends out sound waves. These sound waves bounce back off of the body's internal structures and are detected by the probe. An image is then created using the returning sound waves.

The density of a tissue determines how much the sound waves can penetrate. Variation in the reflection of the sound waves differentiates tissues (muscle, bone, fat, etc.). The ultrasound machine uses this information to create the image. Bone is a very dense tissue and is a barrier to imaging some internal structures through the skin.

Ultrasound of the heart (I'm covering this mostly because it's cool)
Ultrasound of the heart is called *echocardiography*. Many images of your heart are possible using a probe that is placed in specific locations on the outside of the chest. Viewing certain structures in more detail, such as your heart valves, may require a different type of probe that allows viewing from the inside of the body. This test, called *transesophageal echocardiography* (TEE, for short), uses a long probe that is passed through the same path as food you swallow (through your esophagus). This approach gets the probe close to the heart without bone in the way—makes for some impressive images! Don't worry, topical freezing medication is used to numb the throat and sedative medications are generally used to make this procedure more comfortable.

Endoscopy

How It Works
Similar to the long probe used for the TEE procedure described above, endoscopy procedures also use probes to view inside your body. Instead of using ultrasound, these probes have small video cameras at the tip. These cameras allow the surface of body structures to be seen wherever the tip of the probe is inserted. The reason for these tests can range from routine screening to monitoring of a known disease. Freezing and sedatives are thankfully used here too. Common endoscopy tests include:

- Colonoscopy—to examine the inside surface of the colon
- Gastroscopy—to examine the inside of the stomach
- Bronchoscopy—to examine the inside of the lungs

Now, I've included the words "you" and "probe" in the same sentence a couple of times here. Sorry about that. It's possible that it might elicit somewhat of a cringe—perhaps an unconscious tightening of your body… I get that. Ironically, the opposite reaction makes the procedure a lot easier on you. That's where the sedative medications come in—artificial rest and relaxation. Convenient and appealing!

Electrocardiogram (ECG—also referred to as EKG)

This test monitors the electrical activity of your heart.

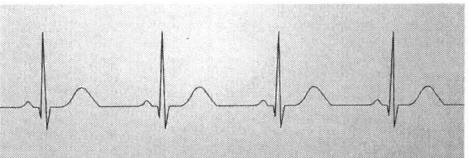

How It Works

Small wires pick up this electrical activity through a connection to small gel-containing stickers (electrodes) that are placed in certain locations around your chest. This electrical activity is then converted and displayed as a waveform on a monitor screen.

In the Operating Room, you'll have an ECG for sure—either with three or five of those electrode stickers with a wire clipped to each of them. For pre-operative testing, you'll have a "12-lead ECG" that uses 10 electrodes. This allows for diagnosis of issues with heart rate and rhythm (called an *arrhythmia* or *dysrhythmia*).

Interpretation of ECG waveforms requires a trained eye. Many abnormal heart conditions can be diagnosed using an ECG and it is one of the most common medical tests. Fortunately, it is also relatively easy to do and causes no discomfort (except when the electrodes are taken off—no fun for the guys with hairy chests).

Pulmonary Function Testing (PFT)

This category of tests is used specifically to diagnose and monitor respiratory (lung) disease and disorders. Ahead of surgery, pulmonary function tests are commonly ordered for patients with known or suspected issues with their lungs and breathing. Most PFTs are performed in dedicated labs that have specialty equipment for performing these tests.

Blood Work

Many surgeries that are considered minor do not require blood tests. However, certain health issues and diseases do require a blood test, even if the surgery is minor. So, if you need it, you need it. The more complex and invasive the surgery, the more likely blood and other testing will be performed.

How It Works
If you haven't had blood taken before, here's the scoop:

- A needle will be placed in the vein (this is the ouch part—hint: don't watch!)

- Glass tubes collect the blood for testing

- The needle is removed, pressure is applied to the site and a bandage is applied

- *Tip: To keep your bruise as small as possible, keep pressure on the site with your finger for a least a few minutes afterwards*

> **INSIDER TIP**
>
> If you happen to feel a little nauseous or light-headed while getting your blood taken, tell someone right away. Don't be embarrassed or try to fight it. This response happens to some people with pain, needles, etc. The fancy name for this is *vasovagal response*. It happens because your parasympathetic nervous system gets a little more active than usual and causes your blood pressure to drop.

CONFESSION
Did you read the Insider Tip above? This happened to me while I was getting blood taken! Ugh. It's a transient experience and fortunately it passes quickly. The usual treatment is just to have the person lay down with their head flat and legs elevated on a couple pillows. I was sitting in a chair at the time and just had to lay my head on the table in front of me for a few minutes. Odds are that it won't happen to you but in case it does, you won't be so caught off guard.

There are many more medical tests out there but these are the most common. They all offer important insights into your health. Your healthcare team will use this information to guide your preparation for surgery, including exercise, diet and medications, so that your health is the best it can be on the day of your surgery.

APPENDIX C
MONITORING IN THE OPERATING ROOM

IN CHAPTER 3, you were introduced to the three essential monitors used for any operation—electrocardiogram, pulse oximeter and blood pressure monitor. For those interested in learning more about these and other commonly used monitors, descriptions of each are listed below. Enjoy!

How to Use This Appendix

I recommend reading at least the first three sections—Electrocardiogram (ECG/EKG), Pulse Oximeter and Blood Pressure Monitor. These monitors are used for all surgeries. If you're interested in learning more, feel free to continue on to the rest (they are important but not vital for you to know).

Electrocardiogram (ECG/EKG)

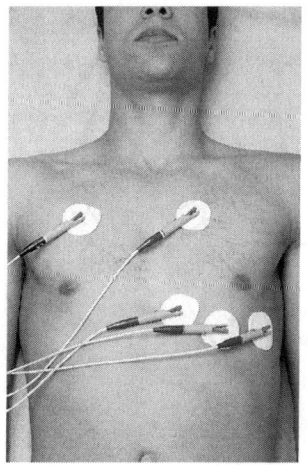

We covered the ECG in Chapter 3 when we talked about pre-operative tests. This is also a standard monitor used in the Operating Room. If you recall, an ECG (also referred to as an ECG) is a monitor that detects and displays the electrical activity of the heart. Here's a picture of how the electrodes and cables will look—close to it, anyway. It is painless and easy to perform, although interpreting an ECG takes expert training.

Pulse Oximeter (Oxygen Saturation Monitor)

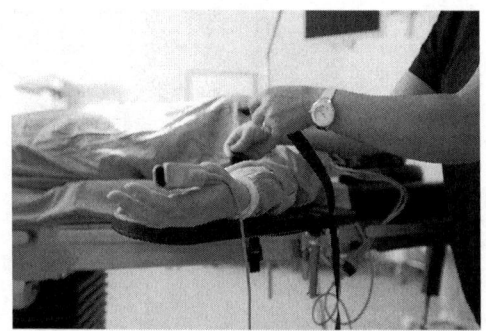

This monitor uses two different wavelengths of light (red and infrared) to determine the amount of oxygen your blood cells are carrying. Red blood cells carrying oxygen absorb these lights differently than those not carrying oxygen. The technology is called pulse oximetry.

The oximetry probe is a small clip that is placed over one of your fingers. You can see the red light if you look closely.

Blood Pressure Monitor

To monitor your blood pressure, a cuff is wrapped around your upper arm that is attached to a small hose. Through this hose, the cuff can be pressurized with air—high enough to stop blood flow past the cuff. As the pressure in the cuff is released, blood begins to pulse past the cuff. This pulsing blood flow creates pressure waves (*oscillations*) detected by the cuff. These pressure oscillations are used to calculate each component of blood pressure—systolic, diastolic and mean. A typical systolic/diastolic blood pressure reading would be $^{120}/_{80}$ mmHg and mean of 70 mmHg (mmHg = millimetres of mercury, a unit of pressure).

Blood pressure can be measured other ways too:

- Manually, using a stethoscope and a manually inflated cuff

- Invasively, using a small catheter inserted directly into an artery, usually in the radial artery (the place you can feel your pulse on the inside of your wrist)

Other Common Monitors

Temperature Monitoring

During surgery it is easy for your body to get cold which increases your risk of infection and the ability for your wound to heal. Temperature probes are used to measure temperature externally on your skin or internally through a body orifice, typically your mouth or nose (put in while you're asleep).

Stethoscope (Who Doesn't Know This One? ... But Who Knows How It Works?)

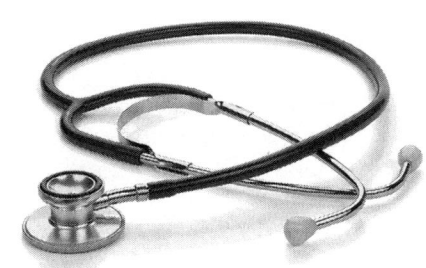

This versatile tool transmits sound from a sensitive diaphragm placed on the skin. These sounds are amplified through a tube and are received by special ear pieces. The key to this technology is that the tube connecting the diaphragm to the ear pieces *amplifies* the sound. As a result, noises are louder and heard more easily by the clinician.

Stethoscopes have a number of uses:

- Manual blood pressure measurement
- Listening to heart sounds
- Listening to lung sounds
- Detecting *bruits* (pronounced *bru-ees*)—these are abnormal "whooshing" sounds caused by blood flowing through narrowed arteries, such as the carotid arteries in your neck

Gas Analysis

Under general anesthesia, you'll breathe a special mixture of gases, containing oxygen and anesthetic gas.

- Gas analysis is used to assess your breathing and measure the amount of anesthetic gas being delivered.

- These are the measured gases:
  - Oxygen (your body's cells need this to live)
  - Carbon dioxide (CO_2—waste gas that you breathe out)
  - Nitrous oxide (an anesthetic gas)
  - Volatile anesthetics (e.g. sevoflurane, desflurane, isoflurane)

Carbon dioxide (CO_2) monitoring is one of the best ways of making sure a patient is breathing properly. As such, CO_2 monitoring is becoming a standard for every patient receiving sedation for a procedure, not just for general anesthesia.

Depth of Consciousness

An interesting fact: your brain's electrical activity changes in fairly predictable ways when you're under general anesthesia. Special monitors have been developed to tell clinicians when changes in your brain waves occur during the anesthetic.

- Depth of consciousness monitoring offers an additional tool to the clinician to assess how deeply asleep you are.

- Monitoring this is easier than you may think! A gel-filled strip of electrodes stuck on your forehead is the only connection required.

Anesthesia Gas Machine & Physiologic Monitor

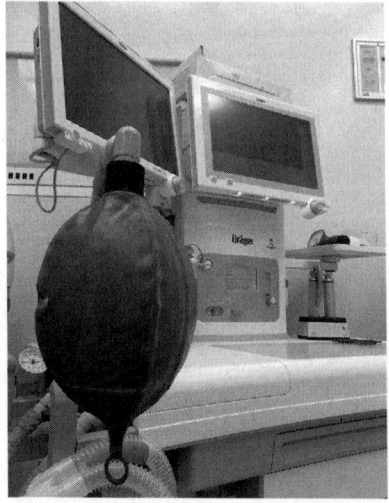

For a general anesthetic, the anesthesia gas machine is used to support your breathing and deliver the anesthetic gases to keep you asleep—it's often the largest piece of equipment in the OR

- Mounted to the anesthesia gas machine, the physiologic monitor does all the hard work of measuring and displaying the ECG, pulse oximetry, blood pressure, temperature and most other monitoring done in the OR

OR Table

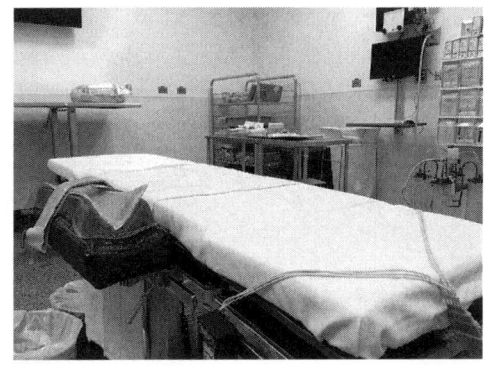

As the name suggests, this more resembles a table than a bed... although this is what you'll be laying on. It is typically narrow, hard and cold.

In some ORs though, the staff are very attentive to making their patients' experience as positive as possible and will place a warmer on the OR table so it is not cold when your bare back touches it. So nice! (I believe this practice should be an expectation—why not take advantage of such an opportunity to help a nervous patient feel comfortable instead of uncomfortable? Ask your team if this is their practice. If it isn't, why not?)

OR Lights

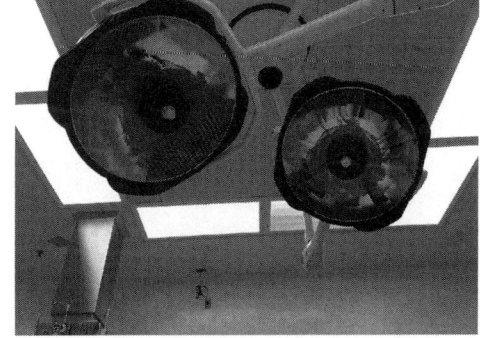

I suppose it's pretty obvious what these are for. But they are quite large and may seem to loom over you as you lay on the OR table. These large discs are sophisticated pieces of engineering that contain dozens of bulbs to create just the right type of illumination in the surgical field—it's good to know the surgeon can see what he or she is doing!

Surgical Equipment

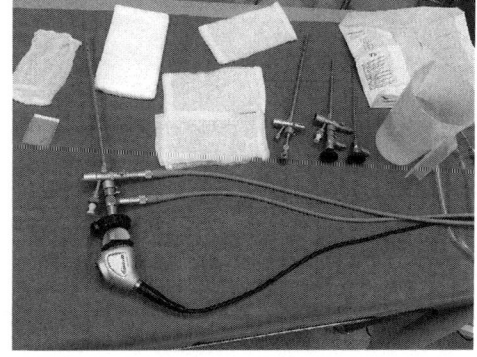

As you enter the OR, you are very likely to see someone standing over a set of instruments. These are the surgical instruments (tools) and the person is the Scrub Nurse, if you recall.

- The Scrub Nurse and the Circulating Nurse together count and document every instrument, gauze and sponge. This is a very important task as this count will be repeated at the end of the surgery to ensure every item is accounted for.

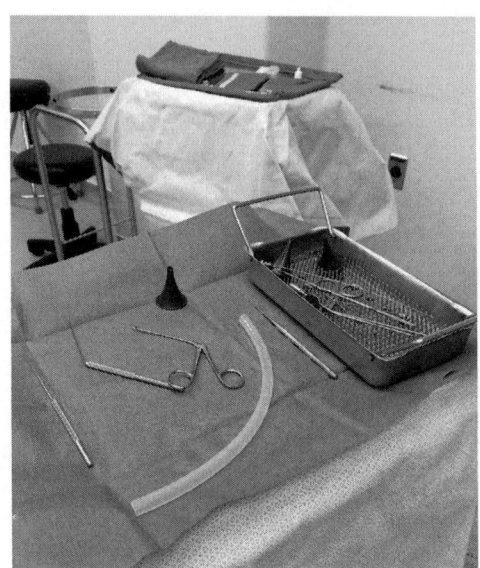

- If there is a discrepancy with the count (meaning that the number of bits counted at the end doesn't match the number they started with), every effort will be made to find what is missing! Most hospitals have a protocol where an x-ray is taken while the patient is asleep if a sponge or instrument is not accounted for.

Monitors, Cameras & Computers

Modern Operating Rooms are often outfitted with technology that allows the Surgical and Anesthesia Teams to access your health records and tests, as well as display, share and record the procedure.

Capturing surgeries digitally is a fantastic tool for professional teaching and collaboration. Rest assured that your permission is required before using any images that may identify you.

A Note About Technology

Above all the technology offering information to the clinician in the OR, the most important thing to attend to is you. A great many things about your status can be appreciated by assessing a patient directly. This is a lesson commonly passed down by experienced clinicians to learners they are mentoring.

APPENDIX D
RESOURCES

DISCOVER THE HOME base for all of our high-quality resources at www.readyformysurgery.com.

Here is a summary of the key resources available to you:

1. **Ready for My Surgery Email Series**

I've compiled a series of short emails with more valuable tips, insights and tools to complement this book. To access this free resource, subscribe at www.readyformysurgery.com.

2. ***Ready for My Surgery* Podcast**

This podcast will connect you with experts in the fields of surgery, anesthesia, pain medicine, rehabilitation as well as other patients. Spend more time than ever before possible listening to healthcare professionals offer you the best advice, tips and wisdom that will help you take action to prepare well, be engaged and optimize your recovery from surgery. Listen anywhere—on the road, at your computer or on your smartphone.

3. Connection Forum
Connect with other patients who have been in your shoes. Find and share support, tips and encouragement. *Who better to give you impressions on surgery than someone who has been through it?*

4. Surveys for the Future
Would you like to contribute to the growth of healthcare delivery? Would you like to see healthcare shaped for patients by the input of patients? By sharing your unique and valuable experience with thousands of other patients through surveys, your voice becomes stronger as themes for change emerge.

5. Other Valuable Resources
Links to other resources that will support your journey through surgery and beyond.

IF YOU HAVEN'T already, continue your journey with me at www.readyformysurgery.com

INDEX

Notes: Page numbers in *italics* denote photos or figures. Page numbers in **bold** refer to the Ready for My Surgery Checklist (Appendix A).

acceptance, 19
acid reflux, 55, 67
Acute Pain Service, 100, 113
    alcohol/recreational substance use, 29, 67, **146**
allergies, 29, **145**
    and blood transfusions, 60; to medications, 115-116
allied health professionals, 46
alveoli, 104
Ambulatory Surgery Centres (ASC), 39-40
anaphylaxis, 115-116
Anesthesia Assistants (AA), 66
Anesthesia Care Team, *64*, 65-66, 68, 70, 83, 86, 119
anesthesiologists, 65
anesthetics, 9-10, 76-77, 79
    and drugs, 29; general anesthesia, 81-83, 85-86, *158*; local anesthetics, 79, 81; lung collapses, 113-114; and memory, 10-11; and nausea/vomiting, 29; recovery from, 10; regional anesthetics, 79-81
anxiety, 17, 67
    and knowledge, xiv; and Operating Rooms, 1, 69; reducing, 2
arrival times, 43, 56
arthritis, 67
artificial airways, 68, 86-88
aspiration, 55
asthma, 22, 67

back/neck pain, 67
bed sores/pressure sores, 106
belongings, 42, **147**
blood clots, 104-105, 114
blood pressure monitoring, 156
blood transfusions, 9, 31, 60, 67, **144**
blood work, 154
breathing support, 124

calls to action
    fears, 20; hospital types, 40; medical tests, 32; night before surgery, 54;

Ready for My Surgery
Checklist, 30, 43
Canada, 98
    listings of family doctors,
    21; quitting smoking, 26
Canadian Patient Safety
    Institute (CPSI), 22
cancer, 67
Cardiovascular Perfusionists, 71
Certified Registered Nurse
    Anesthetists (CRNA), 66
children, and surgery, 28
Choose Wisely campaign,
    32, 33
chronic health issues, 21-22
chronic obstructive pulmonary
    disease (COPD), 22, 67
chronic pain, 89
Circulating Nurse, 70
Clinical Fellows, 45
clotting disorders, 67
communication breakdowns,
    110-111
Community Hospitals, 39, 65
complaining, 135
complex surgeries, 120
Computerized Tomography
    (CT) scan, *150*
consent forms, 61
constructive criticism, 135-137
correct patient, correct site,
    correct procedure, 9, 61-62

deep breathing exercises,
    103-104
delays/cancellations, 10, 39,
    68-69
depression, 67
depth of consciousness monitoring, 158

diabetes, 22, 67, 106
drugs, and anesthetics, 29

echocardiography, 152
electrocardiogram (ECG/EKG)
    tests, *153*, *155*
emergencies, post-surgery,
    111-112
emergency surgeries, 39, 69,
    120, 122
emotions, normalcy of, 19
endoscopy, 152-153
endotracheal tubes, 88
epidural anesthetics, 80
ERAS (Enhanced Recovery
    After Surgery) Society
    guidelines, 22-23, 105
exercise, 113-114, 127-128,
    146-147
    deep breathing, 103-104,
    113-114; getting out of
    bed, 104
experience, sharing, 14
eye surgery, 40

family doctors, 21, 126
    discussing surgery with, 20;
    GP-Anesthetists, 65
family/friends, 50, 84-85,
    95-96, 125-126
fasting, 9, 43, 54-55
feedback/thank yous,
    134-136
feeding tubes, 105

gas analysis, 157-158
general anesthesia, 81-83,
    85-86, *158*
Google, 41, *101-102*
gratitude, 19

hand-washing, 119-120, *121*
health conditions, 67
healthcare teams, xv
heart disease, 22
heart system, 67
high blood pressure, 22, 67
high cholesterol, 67
home, recovery in, 13, 110,
    124-126, **147**
home care/community
    care, 126
hospital administration and
    office staff, 47
Hospital Board of Directors, 47
hospital wards, 97
hospitals, 8
    Ambulatory Surgery
    Centres (ASC), 39-40;
    Community Hospitals,
    39; feedback for, 134;
    feeling lost in, 19; flow
    through, 9, 48-50;
    giving back to, 137-138;
    hospital wards, 97;
    Intensive Care Units,
    13, 49, 120, 122-124;
    navigating, 41; Ready
    for My Surgery Checklist,
    144; recovery in, 11-12;
    University Teaching
    Hospitals, 38-39, 122;
    visitors, 119
hydration, 24, 55

incisions, caring for,
    106-107
infections
    blood transfusions, 60;
    preventing, 106-107,
    119-120, *121*, **147**;
    reducing risks of, 12

insider tips
  blood work, 154; booking surgeries, 68; emergency surgeries, 69; feeling lost, 19; infections/"super bugs," 31; IVs, 78; pain medications, 113; Pre-Operative Area, 49, 61; sedation, 81; smoking, 24-27; students, 71; surgery appointments, 43; University Teaching Hospitals, 38
Intensive Care Units (ICU), 49, 123-124
  recovery in, 13, 120, 122; University Teaching Hospitals, 122
interns, 44
IVs, 10, 60, 77-79, 83

kidney disorders, 67
knowledge, importance of, xiv

liver disease, 67
local anesthetics, 79, 81
lung diseases, 67
lung tissue collapse (atelectasis), 113-114
lungs/respiration, 67

Magnetic Resonance Imaging (MRI), 150, 151
medical doctors, 44-45, 97-100
medical residents, 44-45
medical students, 44, 71
medical tests, 8, 12, 20, 31-32, **145**, 149, 151-154
  Pre-Operative Area, 60-61

medications, 43, **146**
  blood thinners, 105; for pain, 12, 96, 113-116; questions about, 12; side effects/allergies, 115-116, **147**
memory, 67
  and anesthesia, 10-11, 87
mindfulness, 54, 127
monitoring technology, 160
morning of the surgery, 56

nausea/vomiting, 29, 54-55, 81, 88-89
nerve blocks, 80-81
neuromuscular diseases, 67
neuropathy, 67
night before surgery, 9, 53-54
Nurse Practitioners (NPs), 100
nutrition, 23-24, 55, 110, 128, **147**
  post-surgery, 105-106

obesity, 22, 67
Occupational Therapists (OT)/ Occupational Therapist Assistants (OTA), 99
Operating Rooms, 48-49, 69-71, 72, 73, 74, 158-159
  and anxiety, 1, 69; expenses, 68-69; experiences in, 10
opportunity, surgery as, 20
OR lights, 159
OR nurses, 70
OR table, 159
organization, importance of, 28-29, 43
oxygen masks, 83

pain, 127
  communication about, 11-12, 112-113; controlling, 89, 113-117; medications for, 12, 114-115
parents, discussing surgery with children, 28
parking, 42
Parkinson's disease, 67
participation in healthcare, importance of, 18
Patient-Centred Care (PCC), 94-96
patient-controlled analgesia (PCA), 116
patient engagement, importance of, 18
peripheral nerve blocks, 80-81, 116
pharmacists, 99, 126
Physician Assistants (PAs), 99
Physiotherapists (PT)/ Physiotherapist Assistants, 98
planning
  arrival times, 41; getting home, 43; questions to answer, 41-43; routes, 41-42, **144**
Post-Anesthetic Care Unit (PACU), 49, 86, 87, 89, 94
post-surgery tests, 12, 117
post-surgical checklist/Sign Out, 75, 85
Pre-Admission Clinic visits, 8, 30-31, 64, 66, 68, **145**
Pre-Operative Area, 9, 48, 56-59, 61, 70
  Anesthesia Team, 66

pre-surgery appointments, 30-31
pre-surgical checklist/Sign In, 63, 75-76
pregnancy, 67
prescribed exercises, 11-12
pressure sores/bed sores, 106
professional associations, *101-102*
Professional Regulatory Colleges, *102*
Pulmonary Function Testing (PFT), 153-154
pulse oximeter (oxygen saturation monitor), 155, *156*

questions, 8, 32, 41-43
    about medications, 29, 97, 117, *118*; asked in the Pre-Operative Area, 9, 48, 57-59, 66; best time to ask, 49; importance of asking, 20, 59, 68

Ready for My Surgery Checklist, 8, 30, 41-42, 66, 111, 115, 125, **144-148**
recovery, 103-108, 129
    in Hospital Wards, 94, 96; Intensive Care Unit, 13, 120, 122-124; motivation, 127; planning, 103; Ready for My Surgery Checklist, **147**; timeframes, 11; understanding expectations, 18
regional anesthetics, 79-81
Registered Dieticians, 23, 100
Registered Nurses (RNs), 45, 99

Registered Practical Nurses (RPNs), 99
Registered Respiratory Therapists (RRTs), 49, 99, 124
rehabilitation, 127
risks, **144**
    avoidable, xv

sedation, 79-81
seizures, 67
Sign In/pre-surgical checklist, 63, 75-76
Sign Out/post-surgical checklist, 75, 85
skin care, 106
sleep apnea, 22, 67
smoking, 8, 24-27, 67, 127-129, **146**
Social Workers, 100
sore throats, 87-88
specialist referrals, 30
specialists, 98-100
Speech-Language Pathologists (SLPs), 100
spinal anesthetic, 80
Spiritual Care/Chaplains, 100
Staff Physicians, 45
stethoscopes, *157*
stress hormones, effects of, 1
stress responses, 105
strokes, 67
support
    asking for, 28; and family/friends, 50, 95-96
support staff, 46-47
supralaryngeal airways/laryngeal mask airways, 88
surgeons, 45, 61, 70-71, **145**

surgery
    and appearance, 93; asking questions about, 3; author's experience of, 133; complex, 120; day of, **146**; impacts of, 93; Ready for My Surgery Checklist, **144**; talking about, 27
surgical complications, 122, **144**
surgical equipment, *159-160*
Surgical/First Assistant, 71
Surgical Pause/Time Out, 63, 75, 84
Surgical Reception, 48, 56
Surgical Safety Checklist, 10, **144**
Surgical Sign In, 63, 75-76
Surgical Sign Out, 75, 85
Surgical Wards, 49-50
surgical wounds, caring for, 106-107
surveys, 134
swallowing issues, 67

temperature probes, 157
thyroid disorders, 67
Time Out/Surgical Pause, 63, 75, 84
transportation, 28, 42-43, 126

ulcers, 67, 106
ultrasounds, *151*, 152
United States, 98
    listings of family doctors, 21; quitting smoking, 26
University Teaching Hospitals, 38-39
    Intensive Care Units (ICU), 122

unpreparedness, 43

vision/hearing issues, 67
vital signs, 10
   monitoring, 72–75, 84, 155–156
volunteers, 47, 100, 138

Wong-Baker FACES Pain Rating Scale, 112, *113*

World Health Organization Guidelines for Safe Surgery, 62
World Health Organization Surgical Safety Checklist, 75–76
wound dehiscence, 107
wrong-site surgery, 62–63

x-rays, *149*, 150

your appearance, impacted by surgery, 93
your care, aspects you control, 123
your health, **145**
   knowing/understanding, 21; and your role in the surgery team, 62–63

ABOUT THE AUTHOR

PATRICK J. NELLIS is a Registered Respiratory Therapist and Certified Clinical Anesthesia Assistant. Patrick is driven to see patients and their families be well-informed, engaged and confident in making decisions that affect their health and healthcare. He believes that better patient outcomes are achieved when strong connections and meaningful partnerships exist between patients and their healthcare providers. In addition to writing, Patrick enjoys martial arts, rock climbing, travelling and occasionally picking up his guitar. He lives in Georgetown, Ontario, Canada, with his wife and two children.

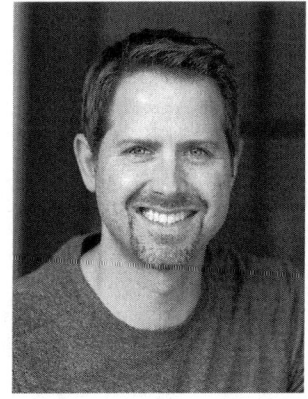

Made in the USA
Monee, IL
03 May 2026

49438429R00109